Also by Rick Lamplugh

In the Temple of Wolves
A Winter's Immersion in Wild Yellowstone

Deep into Yellowstone
A Year's Immersion in Grandeur and Controversy

The Wilds of Aging
A Journey of Heart and Mind

WHAT HELPING PROFESSIONALS SAY ABOUT *THE WILDS OF CANCER*

As a physician, I wish I could prescribe this book. Rick Lamplugh's journey through his treatment of prostate cancer is a masterclass in patient empowerment. With raw honesty, he shares his fears and successes, creating a holistic map for healing that beautifully integrates rigorous research, profound lifestyle changes, and the restorative power of nature. *The Wilds of Cancer* is a must-read for patients seeking not just to survive, but to thrive.

> **KEITH R. HOLDEN**, MD, publisher of *Prostate Cancer Secrets* (Substack)

This is a deeply human love story of how, together, Rick and Mary navigate the twists and turns of Rick's prostate cancer diagnosis and treatment—their curiosity, agility, and openness to adapt resonate with my own caregiving approach. I discovered a soulful and humble flow of life woven within these pages, beautifully in sync with these nature lovers.

> **VICTORIA CHIN**, MBA, founder of *Carer Mentor: Empathy & Inspiration* (Substack)

With the observational skills of a wilderness guide, Rick Lamplugh navigates the profound questions and hard realities of his cancer diagnosis, inviting readers into his most vulnerable moments and ecstatic breakthroughs, all within a compelling framework of helpful information and the powerful blessings of companionship.

> **CAROLINE KRAUS**, author of *Borderlines: A Memoir*, writer and director of the documentary *Moments of Truth*

As both a urologist and fellow patient, I saw myself in these pages. The tough choices, the fear, the unknown. This book captures one man's journey with honesty and grace. It shows how walking in nature can help us breathe, quiet the noise, and bring clarity to hard decisions. And how loved ones can offer strength and hope at the most difficult crossroads.

THOMAS GREEN, MD, publisher of *Urologist with Prostate Cancer* (Substack)

The Wilds of Cancer is just what the doctor ordered! Rick Lamplugh provides the reader with a unique view of cancer from the time of diagnosis through treatment—all from the perspective of the patient.

KENDALL CHILD, Nurse Practitioner

As an oncologist, I see every day how healing depends on more than medicine. Rick Lamplugh captures this truth beautifully in *The Wilds of Cancer*. He brings us into the raw moments of cancer treatment while showing how time outdoors, a steady mindset, and daily practices like diet, rest, and exercise can help carry a person through. This book is both a story and a guide—one that patients, families, and even doctors will learn from.

DANIEL FLORA, MD, PharmD, publisher of *Curative* (Substack)

Thank you for sharing your most challenging of times. I am so very grateful for your strength and resilience in these times. You continue to inspire people to face their challenges and have compassion for themselves and others.

BRENDA PAPERA, RN, BSN

WHAT READERS SAY ABOUT
THE WILDS OF CANCER

The images and feelings really come alive for me in your writing, and my heart goes out to you and Mary.

ALAN KIRK

Love the analogy you make between bison and wolves needing territory to grow their populations and viewing cancer cells as wildlife needing the same. And how that analogy gives you the goal of "starving" them.

BARB KELLY

I am following your journey with love, hope, and a bit of fear.

KATHI WHITSON

The way you describe your journey is so inspiring and powerful. I can feel your pain, your feelings of loss, and your anxiety of not being able to win the battle against cancer. Through your writing, you help others.

ILSE KAPPY

An inspiring story of tribulation, concern, struggling emotions, introspection, and insight.

CHARLES ROTH

Animals have a way of helping us through the funk we are in, whether it would be waking up in a bad mood or helping those with cancer weather the storm. Thank you for sharing your stories of your battle. It puts appreciating life into proper perspective.

DIANE CAIN

I just want to say thank you for sharing your cancer journey with the world. It brought great hope to my husband.

NANCY WARREN

I truly believe this will be a valuable resource for this reason: one man's prostate cancer is another woman's breast cancer is another man or woman's.... pick your cancer. And for those who have never had cancer, everyone knows either a loved one or friend who has. It's part of the universal human dilemma, and none of us is immune.

GREG FIELD

Your book is going to help others navigate suffering.

PAT LOVERME

I wish everyone facing a life-changing event would look around and see how the beauty of nature can help change that funk feeling.

SANDY WEBER

Reading your journey is very compelling, and it's as though I'm standing next to you, watching and feeling everything that you are experiencing.

LAUREN SMITH

The Wilds of Cancer

A Life-Affirming Journey

Rick Lamplugh

This is a work of nonfiction. All quoted material from medical professionals is transcribed from authorized audio recordings. Quoted material from other sources is based on my memories of conversations. I have left out the names of medical professionals to protect their privacy. All other names used are those of real people.

The Wilds of Cancer text copyright 2026 by Rick Lamplugh
Published by: Wild Publishing
Photo of author copyright Mary Strickroth
Front cover photo copyright Mary Strickroth
Cover and interior design: Open Heart Designs

Catalog information: The Wilds of Cancer: A Life-Affirming Journey / Rick Lamplugh. —First Edition

1. Cancer—Prostate Cancer
2. Cancer—Treatment
3. Cancer—Recovery
4. Lamplugh, Rick—Journeys
5. Lamplugh, Rick, 1948-

ISBN (paperback) 979-8-9938154-0-4
ISBN (eBook) 979-8-9938154-1-1

Printed in the United States of America on library-quality stock

10 9 8 7 6 5 4 3 2 1

For Mary, Allison, Zack, Hana, and Siena

Contents

Introduction

The Wilds of Cancer began as journaling—visits to my paper therapist—after I was diagnosed with aggressive prostate cancer. That diagnosis surprised me, scared me, and sent me into a whirlwind of wild thoughts, emotions, and moments as my wife, Mary, and I struggled to cope. Eventually, we met the challenge of researching and choosing treatment: forty-four shots of radiation and eighteen months of hormone therapy. As treatment progressed, I had to learn how to deal with significant side effects and life changes.

During almost two years of troubling times brought on by cancer, I fluctuated between wanting and not wanting to turn my journal entries into a book. I had successfully done this with two previous books, *In the Temple of Wolves* and *The Wilds of Aging*. Both won awards and were widely read. So why was I struggling with whether to publish *The Wilds of Cancer*?

Sometimes I rationalized that I was too busy to bother with bringing out a book. At other times, I wondered whether I had the courage to share such a personal story, especially if treatment failed and my cancer spread.

That struggle came to a head during the summer when Mary and I reached our second summit of the season. This one was 10,300 feet, and the four-mile trail to the summit was a killer. The steeper-than-steep last half-mile pushed me close to my limits. Not just a physical limit, but also a mental limit. I even said aloud to one of my hiking partners, "I don't know if I can do this." She kept pushing on, providing a good example. I kept mumbling my discontent, but I followed.

When we reached the top, the view and the feeling of accomplishment were grand. As I sat on the rocky summit, gobbling a sandwich and guzzling water, I thought of how that hike was a metaphor for my battle with cancer: a long, challenging journey that I sometimes thought I couldn't do, wouldn't finish. But sitting there, months after the successful treatment had ended, my view of the future and my sense of accomplishment were grand, and helped me decide to publish.

I'm glad you decided to read this book. Each chapter will focus on my long journey into the wilds of cancer. While I'll touch on my months of effective and conventional medical treatment, these are not stories about how to medically treat cancer. I'm a writer, not a doctor, and I'm not offering medical advice.

I'll share stories about how, after the diagnosis, Mary and I found ways to handle an onslaught of facts and feelings and lifestyle changes as we sought the most positive way, the most hopeful way, the most life-affirming way, to face a frightening and seemingly unending challenge in our lives.

I hope you'll find much to relate to in these honest and heartfelt stories of our journey into the wilds of cancer.

CHAPTER 1

Into the Wild

O<small>N THE SUMMER SOLSTICE AND OUR WEDDING ANNIVER-</small>sary, Mary and I were hiking with our friend Fred. While climbing a steep hillside in a national forest, we stopped to catch our breath and watch some female elk and their young watch us. The young had lost their spotted coats, but their mothers had not lost their protective nature. We kept our distance and shared the joy of this wild moment. Thankful, we resumed walking through knee-high grass dotted with colorful wildflowers.

Until the ringing of my cell phone shattered the wild silence.

I usually kill the phone when I hike, but I was awaiting a call from my urologist with the results of a prostate biopsy. I glanced at the phone's screen; it was him. I felt relief and dread. I would finally know the results. They might be bad.

"I have to take this," I said. Mary jerked her head toward me, concern obvious. She knew about the call. I gave her a nod. As I turned away, Mary and Fred silently looked at each other and found a seat on a couch-sized boulder left by a melting glacier at the end of the last ice age. I walked a few paces, took a deep breath, and put the phone on speaker. Nerves tingling, I managed a little small talk.

The urologist quickly moved to the heart of the matter: "Unfortunately, we did find cancer..."

My shoulders sagged, and my stomach tightened as he described how the biopsy revealed prostate cancer cells with varied degrees of aggressiveness. One set of cells was not very aggressive. One was medium aggressive. But a very aggressive third set concerned him. And that concerned me.

He recommended a nuclear bone scan to see if the cancer had spread to my bones. Spread to my bones? I didn't like the sound of that, but I agreed to the scan, and we clicked off.

I looked at my hiking partners. Mary made eye contact. I shook my head from side to side. Her face registered shock and sadness as her head sank. I walked over and stood silent, struggling to deliver news I didn't want to believe, let alone repeat. Finally, I said, "The biopsy found cancer in my prostate."

Fred said softly with sad eyes, "Rick, I'm so sorry to hear that."

Without a word, Mary moved to me. We hugged, and I found solace in the warmth of her neck, the softness of her shoulder-length hair, and the rustle from the wings of a raven flying overhead.

The three of us stood speechless on that hillside under a big, blue Montana sky speckled with clouds. Trying to distract myself, I looked for the elk, but they had moved on. Instead, I studied a nearby line of snow-streaked crags in Yellowstone National Park and felt the discord of receiving ugly news in a beautiful place. We returned to the car. That hike was over; a new journey had begun.

Mary told me later that she had heard the doctor describe the very aggressive cancer. With tears in her blue-gray eyes, she said, "I don't want to lose you, Rick. I don't want to find out what it means to live without you."

I held her and trembled as I felt my deep love and longing for her. I told her I didn't want our time together to end, either. We had been friends for fifty years, partners for twenty-four, and married for nineteen.

It wasn't just Mary I wanted more time with. I longed to see the lives of our two kids and their partners unfold as they approached midlife. I hoped to see our granddaughter finish school and continue exploring her talents. And I wanted more years with friends experiencing wild moments in wild lands.

While ten or twenty more years didn't seem like a lot, I feared that might not happen.

CHAPTER 2

Our First Guide

UNKNOWINGLY, I BEGAN THIS JOURNEY INTO THE WILDS of cancer well before I received my diagnosis. Two months earlier, Mary and I were on a guided rafting and hiking trip through the Grand Canyon. The guide was essential. We lacked the skills to handle the ever-changing water conditions and were unfamiliar with the trails we hiked on. The guide gave us direction and reassurance.

While the guided days were fun, the nights in the canyon were troubling. I awoke so many times to urinate that I wondered what was wrong. The nighttime busyness continued in a motel after the trip ended. Concerned, I recorded my liquid input and output for several days and took the records to a scheduled annual exam with my primary care doctor once we returned home to Montana. I discussed the data and my worries with her. She ordered urine and blood labs. The urine lab showed no irregularities. But the blood work revealed the PSA score that started this journey.

PSA stands for prostate-specific antigen, a protein produced by normal — and malignant — prostate gland cells. A PSA score is measured in nanograms per milliliter, but is usually abbreviated to just the number. Most doctors look for a PSA of four or higher when deciding whether to test for prostate cancer. My score was twenty-five.

That high score shocked me into researching PSA testing. I was surprised to learn that my doctor could have justified *not testing*. I found a section of the American Urological Association website that presented a prostate cancer curriculum for medical students and described varying accepted standards. One stated that men over seventy and in excellent health may benefit from testing. Another recommended *no testing* for any men seventy and older. Since I was seventy-three, I was thankful to have a primary care doctor who requested a PSA test, studied the results, and referred me to my first urology consult. Mary immediately volunteered to accompany me. I treasured her willingness to attend, listen, and question, as we could have different takeaways from deep discussions.

When we walked into that initial urology consult, I yearned to find a guide for this journey into unknown territory. I was determined to ask the urologist where he stood on treating prostate cancer in "a man my age." In the last few years, I had grown to dislike that expression, but it fits.

Before we began, I asked the urologist, "Can I record our conversation?"

"That's a good idea," he said. He went on to explain that prostate cancer can be found in up to seventy-five percent of men my age and older. My lack of symptoms was expected. He would typically not see symptoms until the cancer was far advanced. With my high PSA score, he gave me a fifty-fifty chance of having prostate cancer.

He asked if I had had PSA tests during previous annual exams. He wanted to establish a baseline or identify changes in the PSA number over time. A rise could increase the odds that I had active cancer cells in my prostate and that further testing was needed. As I explained that I had been healthy my entire adult life and rarely visited doctors, I finally admitted to myself that missing numerous annual exams and PSA tests was a mistake. I knew Mary would agree: she had repeatedly encouraged me to have PSA tests over the years.

I told the urologist I had read that treatment for prostate cancer was not always recommended for men over seventy. He said the current thinking was that men my age had so few years left to live on average that something else would likely take us before prostate cancer. Testing and treatment, which can be expensive and have troublesome side effects, might not be necessary.

He gestured toward me with his tattooed arm. "But look at you, you're physically fit, not overweight, and on no medications. You have a good ten to twenty years left. Why not treat you?"

I smiled and silently calculated that perhaps I could have more years with Mary, our family, and our friends.

A statistic I uncovered boosted this hope: while prostate cancer was common, of those diagnosed, only about one man in six died from the disease. Five of six didn't. I could live, no pun intended, with those odds.

The urologist said that an accurate diagnosis required a biopsy. He would take samples from my prostate and send them to a lab that would determine if cancer cells were present and how aggressive they were. He would call me with the results. I agreed to schedule a biopsy appointment.

As the initial consult ended, I realized we had found our first guide. He would be as essential as the guide who led us through the Grand Canyon. Mary and I needed guidance in handling the ever-changing medical information. We did not know the medical trail we would travel or how long we would be on it. We would look to this guide, and perhaps others, for direction and reassurance.

CHAPTER 3

Return to Journaling

THIS JOURNEY INTO THE WILDS OF CANCER WAS FILLED with scary possibilities. The biggest, of course, was that this disease would kill me. My days post-diagnosis were often a battle between the fear that I would die and the hope that I wouldn't.

To make matters worse, I had no idea how long this journey would be. However long, I knew I had to be honest with myself. This would not be just a battle to protect my body. This would also be a journey of heart and mind. My heart would open to many feelings about facing and perhaps falling to cancer. My mind would search for facts, for ways to treat and beat the disease. I expected an onslaught of facts and feelings. Both would be important, work well together, and help me make decisions.

I would deal with that onslaught by honest journaling each morning, an approach that had helped me through a previous troubling time.

I had just turned sixty and was on a 375-mile solo bicycle tour. I had been on other challenging tours, but never alone. My usual riding partner had to pull out at the last minute. While cycling in Washington's North Cascades, I felt, for the first time, that I had hit an impenetrable wall. I didn't have the strength, energy, or gumption to continue climbing in full sun up a steep, hot grade toward a mountain pass that seemed to keep sneaking away. And I didn't have any riding partners to help me cope.

I pulled off the road, dropped my bike, and stumbled down a rocky slope to a stream. I spent the next hour dipping my head into the cold stream and debating, sometimes aloud, whether to retreat or advance. Finally, I removed my shirt and submerged it. Without wringing it out, I pulled it on, shivered, felt refreshed, and chose to keep going. When I reached the pass, I made camp and gave myself a quiet and proud pat on the back as I crawled, exhausted, into my tent.

Though I finished the tour, that scary moment jolted me into journaling for a year in our peaceful backyard garden in Corvallis, Oregon, where we lived at the time. As the summer sun gave way to fall rain and winter snow, I sat under a poplar tree and wrote—for the first time—about aging and how my body, mind, heart, and life were changing. Some sessions led to wiping away tears, others to raising a fist in celebration. I came to call this honest journaling of my thoughts and feelings "visiting my paper therapist." Those entries eventually became the core of my last book, *The Wilds of Aging.*

As I entered the wilds of cancer, I knew I had to return to journaling. I journaled on the deck of our home in Gardiner, Montana, at the north gate of Yellowstone National Park. I wrote about my hope that I could beat this disease. I wrote about my fears that I couldn't and that my days were numbered. I wrote about how changes in my body brought about by the cancer or treatment could make life harder for Mary and me. I wrote about our findings as we immersed ourselves in researching treatment, side effects, and outcomes. I wrote about medical consults and milestones.

I had my first medical milestone, a CT scan, a few days after the annual exam that started me on this journey. The CT, which creates images of bones and soft tissues, showed no evidence that cancer had spread. I felt relieved, but the thought that the CT scan did not provide the complete picture lurked in the back of my mind and frightened me. So, I worried and waited for the next milestone, the urologist-recommended nuclear bone scan, which could provide a more definitive look.

If that second scan confirmed that the cancer had not spread, we would know what we were battling and could decide on treatment. If we chose removal of my prostate, surgery could happen within weeks. If we went with radiation of the prostate instead, that would take months to complete.

Maybe in about four months, by my birthday in mid-November, I would see the whole treatment picture. Maybe not. Either way, I had lots of visits to my paper therapist ahead.

CHAPTER 4

Seeking Support

I KNEW MARY WOULD HELP ME FACE MY FEARS ON THIS journey. She would support me as I would support her. But I didn't want her to carry all the burden. I wanted to find others to help me — and us.

I figured a good starting point for me would be to seek out, talk with, and learn from survivors of prostate cancer and other life-changing illnesses. How did they deal with their emotional challenges? How did they find support?

My first conversation, just a week after diagnosis, was a phone call with a friend who had dealt with Parkinson's disease for years. I told her about my cancer diagnosis, the shock, the denial. She recalled feeling both after her diagnosis. We talked more, and she later sent me an email detailing her experience.

"Overwhelmed with feelings of shock, denial, and grief," she wrote, "sharing the news about my diagnosis felt like a daunting task. I told my immediate family right away but held off telling others. I wanted to first come to terms with having Parkinson's, so I would feel less vulnerable to the reactions of others. I also didn't want to be defined primarily as a person with Parkinson's. And finally, I didn't want to be discriminated against—viewed as less able to contribute at work, for example—because I had Parkinson's. Eventually, I started telling others on a need-to-know basis. Looking back, I see that telling others made the diagnosis real, forcing me to move past my denial.

"I had mixed reactions from people I told and an aha moment. Some made unhelpful comments. 'That's terrible.' 'My uncle died of Parkinson's.'

"But the conversation shifted when one friend asked, 'What is that like for you?' I felt completely supported and benefited from sharing what living with the disease meant."

Reading her email, I craved finding people who asked a question like that. I also wondered, for the first time, if my having cancer would change how people saw me. Would I be perceived as less capable of making a contribution? Another fear emerged.

I also thought about denial and its place in dealing with the grief of facing a life-threatening illness. Denial is understandable, even predictable, according to the late author and psychiatrist Elisabeth Kübler-Ross. She described five stages of grief: denial, anger, bargaining, depression, and acceptance.

I first learned of these stages after her book, *On Death and Dying*, was published years ago. I studied them along the way to receiving a bachelor's degree with a concentration in psychology. The validity of these stages has withstood the test of time with slight modifications. Today's view is that the stages need not happen in a strict order, and not every grieving person will experience all five.

I entered denial immediately. I didn't want to repeat to my hiking partners the diagnosis the doctor had given in that phone call I received while we were hiking in the national forest. Repeating the diagnosis would make it real. Whenever the reality of having cancer would pop into my head, I would stop whatever I was doing and mutter, *"This can't be happening to me."* More denial.

I added anger, saying to myself: *"Damn it, this isn't fair! Why do I have cancer? I don't want to face my mortality again!"* I struggled to write and speak that potentially damaging anger out of my body. Sometimes, the visits to my paper therapist succeeded. At other times, the anger remained, and I had to be careful not to dump it on Mary or some other innocent bystander.

I also bargained for a better outcome, proclaiming, *"So I've got cancer. But if I do everything I can to help my body, I'll survive. Won't I?"* While my desire to do everything was genuine, I didn't yet know how to help my body, mind, or heart. I hadn't even chosen a treatment. I had little to bargain with.

I feared I might dip into dark depression and suffer in sadness as my body and life changed. I might be brought low by the reality that I wouldn't live to see our kids hit mid-life or our granddaughter enter adulthood. What could I do to avoid or fight depression?

On better days, I hoped I would live to eventually accept whatever reality prostate cancer created. Days when I would tell myself and others, "I've got prostate cancer. Now it's time to get on with life, to accept this new reality of good days, bad days, dark days, light days." But I didn't know when—or if—that would happen.

Understanding the stages of grief was one thing. Living through them would be another, and I knew I would need to find others to hold my emotional hand.

CHAPTER 5

A Yellowstone Lesson

EARLY IN THIS JOURNEY, I REALIZED I NEEDED TO BE PATIENT; I needed to be *a patient*. I needed to wait for appointments and advice, tests and treatment, recovery and return to normality. If life ever returned to pre-diagnosis normal. Such a monstrous fear. If cancer didn't take me, it might change me in ways I didn't like but couldn't undo.

Still, I was an impatient patient. Though that earlier CT scan had revealed no evidence that cancer had spread, I drummed my fingers while waiting for the nuclear bone scan that could provide a more definitive look and possibly end this seemingly endless struggle to choose treatment. If the scan showed no spread, I could choose between surgery and radiation and get started. If the scan showed spread, Mary and I would begin an even scarier journey with other treatment choices. I knew that as I waited for the scan results, I would waste days wondering and worrying.

But I didn't want to get ahead of myself either. There were too many unknowns and blind spots to look too far down this trail into the wilds of cancer. Perhaps I could better navigate by comparing this unknown trail to something I knew: a lengthy, multi-day trek into Yellowstone's wild backcountry.

Mary and I moved to Gardiner, at Yellowstone's north entrance, soon after we retired. Excited and sad, we thrust ourselves from Corvallis, Oregon, our home for thirty-six years. We were drawn to a place where we loved spending time in the backcountry and had worked, volunteered, and lived seasonally.

During our three winters of working and living at Yellowstone's Lamar Buffalo Ranch, I wrote a book, *In the Temple of Wolves*, about park wolves. When that book was well-received, I realized I owed the wolves a debt. If they could help me, I could help them. I would become an advocate for them. To succeed in this life change, I wanted to learn as much as I could about wolves. I wanted to live where they howled and hunted. I wanted to watch packs and pups. Yellowstone called.

Those winters at the ranch were life-changing for Mary, too. She came away longing to live near and hike in Yellowstone with its wolves and coyotes, elk and bison, bears and mountain lions. She wanted to live, she proclaimed, in a place with more wildlife than people.

With Yellowstone calling, we moved to Gardiner, determined to spend more time backpacking in the park and the surrounding national forest while we were still capable. Once residents, we saw how Gardiner sat at the heart of various environmental issues. I wrote my next book, *Deep into Yellowstone,* about those issues and our adventures in the park.

When we backpacked in and around Yellowstone, I started each day fresh and excited about what lay ahead. I was prepared and present, paying attention to sights, sounds, and sensations. But by afternoon, I was often tired and future-focused. When would we make camp? Would I meet the challenges of the days to come? When would this journey end? But that was wasted worry. I learned that by staying present and staying the course, I always met the challenges and reached the end, no matter what a day brought. So it might be, I hoped, with traveling into the unknown wilds of cancer.

I knew this wouldn't be easy. There would be days when I journaled and shared facts and feelings with my paper therapist. But on other days, fear, anger, and uncertainty would engulf me. I would wonder if I could survive or doubt that I could. I might want to deny reality, not journal or talk about it. Then a new day would begin. Repeat, repeat, repeat until I reach the end of this journey — whenever and whatever that would be.

CHAPTER 6

Tears and Fears

THE DAY HAD FINALLY ARRIVED. THREE WEEKS AFTER MY diagnosis, Mary and I drove to a distant facility for that much-anticipated nuclear bone scan. I wanted the scan to confirm that my prostate cancer had not spread, and I could choose surgery or radiation, stop wondering and worrying, and start treating. If it revealed spread, I had no idea what I would do.

After Mary dropped me off at the clinic's front door, she went looking for parking. I found a private corner in the waiting area and settled in. I wondered if I would sit and think about falling to cancer as I had during the two-hour drive. Those thoughts had brought me to tears. I wanted privacy if more tears came.

Before I started crying, a young technician found me. Through our COVID-required masks, we chatted as we walked down a hall toward the treatment room. She stopped at the bottom of a small set of stairs and asked, "Do you have any problems with going up steps?"

I was startled; I thought of all the hikes I've taken up mountains, including the four we see from the dining room window in our home at Yellowstone's north gate. I wanted to shout, *I enjoy hiking up mountains, for God's sake.*

Then I realized she was asking an appropriate question for "a man my age." And I had better get used to such questions; I wasn't getting any younger. In fact, I was going through this medical wilderness to increase my chances of getting older. I thanked her for inquiring and assured her I would not have problems. Up we went.

Down the hall, we stopped in front of an oversized door with a sign that held me spellbound: CAUTION RADIOACTIVE MATERIALS IN USE. My stomach fluttered with fear; I was there to have a radioactive substance injected into my body. We entered, and the technician calmed me, injected me, and reminded me to return after lunch for the scan.

I exited the clinic, and Mary drove us to where willows and tall conifers bordered a stream that bisected a large city park. We grabbed our lunch cooler, followed the stream, found a shaded bench, and made ourselves at home. After lunch, Mary invited me to lay my head on her lap. As I listened to the stream's babbling and drifted off, I realized again that I was a lucky man. I hoped my luck held.

Back at the clinic, the same tech walked me to the same room and had me lie on the narrow, padded table of the scan machine. After she positioned my body, the table began creeping into the machine. I shut my eyes, listened to the machine whir, and ordered myself to relax.

Afterward, the tech confided that she saw no spread. But she added that the final call was up to the clinic's doctor. I felt a wave of relief and thanked her for easing my fear and worry while I awaited the word.

I left the clinic and slipped into our car. As Mary drove toward the exit, I said, "It's clear."

She studied the intersection ahead and appeared to think I was referring to traffic.

"The *scan* was clear," I said.

She looked at me; her hand rushed to her open mouth. "The scan is clear?"

"Yep."

"Oh, that's wonderful!" She returned her gaze to the road and began to cry. Her tears surprised me. While the news relieved me, I wasn't crying. Why not?

As Mary drove us home, I texted the good news to family and friends, exchanging loving words and happy icons. The next day, at home, I went into my office, logged into my online medical chart, and read the official result: no spread. I also found some unfamiliar medical terms and researched them. I clicked on a Mayo Clinic page and read that if prostate cancer spreads to the bones, there is currently no curative treatment. There are ways to reduce symptoms and prolong life, but there's no way to stop the progression to death.

No cure? Death? Shocked, I called for Mary, who was in her music studio down the hall. When she arrived, she stood beside me and placed a hand on my shoulder. I read her the troubling passage.

"Uh-huh. I knew that," she said. "Didn't you?"

"No, I'm embarrassed to say I didn't." I pulled her hand to my lips, kissed it, started to cry, and whispered, "Now I understand why you cried when I told you the scan was clear."

CHAPTER 7

Our Guide's View

WITH THE CT SCAN AND NUCLEAR BONE SCAN RESULTS finally in, Mary and I needed to meet again with the urologist, our first guide on this journey. Three weeks post-diagnosis, we wanted our guide's view of the trail ahead. We wanted to know what the scans told him and what to expect with radiation or surgery.

When we began the consult, the urologist again approved my recording the session. He stated that with the two scans showing no spread, my cancer "appears to be" confined to the prostate. His qualifier concerned me just as I would be concerned if I asked a guide about the trail we were using to hike up a mountain, and the guide said, "We appear to be on the right trail." Given some of the trails we've taken up and down mountains, I prefer something more definitive.

But I kept my mouth shut as he said that since the cancer hadn't spread, "This is the opportunity that we have to step in and treat your cancer and cure your cancer and thereby save your life." I liked the definitiveness of "cure" and "save."

The urologist explained how cancer works. "Cancer is mutated tissue. And it's mutated in such a way that it acts cancerous; it grows without checks or balances. The more mutated those cells look under a microscope, the more aggressive they tend to behave." He recalled that the lab found cancer in half of my biopsy samples. One sample was rated aggressive and high-risk.

Moving on to possible treatment options, he grabbed a notepad and jotted a short list. He drew a line through "active surveillance," the first item. Active surveillance involves monitoring with PSA tests and biopsies, but does not involve treatment until measurable cancer cell growth is detected. He said this option was out because I had high-risk cancer. I didn't like the sound of that. He said the two remaining options on the list—surgery and radiation—were very different in terms of logistics and side effects. "But they are about equally good."

I listened carefully as he explained that while radiation came in several forms, only external beam radiation was available locally. External radiation of the prostate had side effects. There could be tissue damage to the nearby bladder and rectum. Both could become irritated, and that could cause more urgent and frequent urination, painful bowel movements, and blood in my urine or feces.

"So if I'm looking at painful side effects of treatment, what happens if I do nothing?"

He hesitated, looked down at his paper for a moment, and then into my eyes and said, "The cancer would spread and kill you."

Oh, wrong answer, I thought. "How long?"

"That's a very good question, and I can't answer that. But it's a ticking time bomb, and I would expect you to not be alive in ten years if you do not treat the cancer." Then he asked, "Are you going to be alive in ten years?"

"Well, I'm seventy-three," was all I could come up with as I grappled with the concepts of side effects if I treated and death if I didn't.

"The fact that you already made it to seventy-three," he said, "means you're going to live longer than the average man." He referred to actuarial tables, said I could live twenty more years, and added, "I would not have recommended a biopsy if I thought you had less than a ten-year lifespan."

He moved on to the other treatment option, the surgery he would perform: robotic radical prostatectomy. Radical meant removing the prostate. Robotic meant using an instrument called the DaVinci Robot. He would make a small incision above my belly button and insert a tiny camera and four other instruments. He would control them with the help of the robot. As he moved his fingers, demonstrating how he would manipulate the minuscule instruments, he appeared to be playing a video game. I figured he was young enough to have grown up playing them. That reassured me.

I asked how many of these surgeries he had performed. Although I felt uncomfortable asking, our research indicated that the doctor's relevant experience was essential to successful treatment, whether it involved surgery or radiation. Without hesitation, he said about 150.

He added that surgery had side effects, too: everybody had some urinary leakage after surgery. The leakage usually tapered to the point of requiring only one incontinence pad per day.

"So," I concluded, "one way or the other—radiated or removed—I will have side effects."

He nodded and said that about half the men with prostate cancer choose radiation, and about half choose surgery. Studies show that the overall quality of life at ten years for both groups was about equal. "I would not talk you out of surgery, and I would not talk you out of radiation."

As I silently appreciated his willingness to guide me yet let me choose, he added that I didn't have to make a decision that day. "You'll do some research. You'll talk to each other. You'll talk to friends and family, and you'll choose something that feels right to you. But it's going to come down to a gut feeling. That's all I can tell you."

At that moment, all I felt in my gut was the strain of stress. I was glad to have a few days to digest all this information and ponder. I would also have a radiation consult and perhaps find another guide. The process of choosing a treatment continued to be filled with facts and feelings to face.

CHAPTER 8

Reeling and Stewing

THANKFULLY, MARY DROVE US HOME FROM THE DAUNTING
meeting with the urologist. I was too preoccupied to drive.
By the time we arrived home, I was still a mess. I felt like
I was at a critical point on a long backcountry hike. I had
approached a planned stream crossing and found it raging
and unfordable. I had to decide whether to bushwhack
along the stream in hopes of finding a crossing; search for
an alternative route that avoided the stream; or give up,
turn back, and retrace the miles of hiking I had already
done. None of the options appealed. The stream's awe-
some power made me feel small, vulnerable, and scared.

All day long, the urologist's descriptions of side effects
kept popping into my head, generating scary images of how
my life would change. As the day wore on and the images
wore me out, I emitted long, loud sighs. Traipsing down
the hall, staring out the window, sitting at the desk. Sigh.
Sigh. Sigh. What path, what treatment, do I choose? How
harmful will those side effects be? Should I just give up?

After dinner, Mary encouraged me to share what was in my heart and on my mind, but I didn't want to talk. We watched a comedy on TV, and I chuckled occasionally. Mostly, I drifted in and out of troubling consult replays.

When we went to bed, Mary snuggled against me, settled her head on my chest, and asked, "What are you thinking or feeling right now?"

I appreciated her loving persistence and pushed myself to open up. I groaned and blurted, "That consult was a hell of a shot of reality. I'm struggling to face the reality that I have cancer, that my life is going to be way different."

She raised her head and looked into my eyes. "You're still processing. But remember what the doctor said. The treatment is curative. You're going to live."

The sun was still sleeping when I slipped out of bed the next morning. I fixed a coffee and headed to the deck, ready to journal. The darkness comforted me, and I turned on our little fountain for its mellow murmur. I wore a headlamp with a red beam that lit the journal page but also allowed me to peer into the darkness, spotting clouds and stars, silhouettes, and shadows.

As usual, I had no agenda when beginning a visit with my paper therapist. I started writing, knowing that facts and feelings would follow. I began with the doctor's word: curative. I journaled about my hope that the doctor was correct, my fear that he wasn't, and how my life would change either way.

By the time I finished, the sun was awake and full on me. I closed my journal and headed inside. After breakfast, I moved to the computer to transcribe portions of the recording I had made with the urologist's permission. Transcribing helped me hear things I had missed and generated questions to research. I listened and pondered and typed again and again. By lunchtime, all I wanted was to eat and let the fountain's bubbling and the day's warmth lull me to sleep on a reclined lawn chair on the now-shaded deck.

When I awoke, I returned to transcribing until I heard Mary arrive home from her appointments. She had promised to listen to the consult while driving around, another benefit of recording. I found her, and we began discussing treatment options. I quickly realized that with the day's journaling, transcribing, and discussing, I'd had enough cancer time. I explained this to Mary; I was relieved she understood.

We shifted to pleasant chatter about the plants growing in the backyard. We enjoyed the songs of birds hidden in the trees. We listened and watched an afternoon thunderstorm envelop 10,969-foot Electric Peak. As I felt the day's challenges losing power, I realized that being in and paying attention to nature, whether in the backyard or on the trail, was medicine to me—felt curative. I didn't yet understand how nature helped my body, mind, and heart. But I was thankful for the healing.

CHAPTER 9

Roller Coaster

A TROUBLING MONTH HAD DRAGGED BY SINCE DIAGNOSIS, and we had still not selected a treatment. Yesterday, Mary tried to get me to talk about the options, but I just felt too overwhelmed.

After a good night's sleep, I was finally ready. Mary and I met on the deck for what we call a business meeting. The day's business was surgery versus radiation: remove or radiate. We dove in, discussing facts and sharing feelings. There was so much to consider; I quickly wilted back to overwhelmed, again desperate to stop thinking and talking, wondering and worrying.

While Mary spoke, I drifted away, staring at the trees and shrubs we had planted and nurtured in our backyard over the years. I marveled at their health and growth — except for one, a pine she claimed was dying. I refused to accept that.

A few days earlier, while in the yard by myself, I had gently brushed away some of the pine's dead brown needles and whispered, "I won't give up on you. I'm going to give you every chance to get better."

Then, yesterday, as we had strolled through the yard, touching and speaking to what we call "our green friends," Mary had pointed to the pine and asked, "When do you want to take that out? It's clearly…"

I cut her off. "Let's not say that. I wouldn't go up to a friend and tell him he looks like he's dying."

Her sad and quizzical stare had made me wonder if my response to the ailing pine might represent my emotional struggle with the possibility of dying from cancer. Could be.

On the deck, Mary pulled me from my pining by asking, "You're about done, aren't you?"

"Yeah," I muttered, "I can't believe how overwhelming these decisions are."

She nodded but wasn't ready to stop. "If you had to choose today, what would it be?"

"Surgery. But I might change my mind after the radiology consult."

"I'm in a similar place," she said, smiling.

I put my arm around her, pulled her toward me, and whispered, "Thank you so much for helping me through this."

"Of course! You're not alone."

I kissed her on the cheek and retreated into the house, wondering about other ways this journey into the wilds of cancer would challenge my body, mind, and heart.

Whatever was ahead, I planned to get my body into the best shape for the battle. I walked to the bedroom, set up the dumbbells, and began a strength-and-stretch routine I aim to do twice a week. Forty-five minutes later, I felt refreshed and made a decision: I would schedule surgery to remove my prostate. I would also keep the option to change my mind and choose radiation after the oncology consult.

I strode down the hall to my office, called the urologist, and got on his surgery schedule. One decision down. Plenty to go.

Feeling energized, I decided to make another phone call. A friend had given me the number of another man with prostate cancer and said that this stranger was my age and would talk with me. Nervous about intruding but determined to learn how others handled cancer, I called. He said he had been expecting my call, and we dove into sharing our stories.

Two and a half years ago, his biopsy showed non-aggressive cancer, and he began active surveillance. A year later, another biopsy revealed very aggressive cancer. Waiting was out; treatment was in. He met with a surgeon who warned him that if his prostate was removed, he would be incontinent and might need to wear pads for the rest of his life because of pre-existing issues in his core. He then consulted with a radiologist who described how radiation had become more targeted and had fewer long-term side effects. He chose radiation and two months ago began treatment.

After we wished each other the best in our journeys and ended the call, I stared out the window and realized that, of everything we had discussed, I was most troubled by the image of wearing pads for incontinence. I had faced subtle urination challenges for years, and they'd come to a head on that Grand Canyon vacation when the urge to purge awoke me far too many times each night. Once back home, the blood work ordered by my primary care doctor revealed my PSA score of twenty-five, a number far too high to ignore, which led to a biopsy that led to the diagnosis. Facing prostate cancer knocked my urination worries right out of the picture.

But the discussion about wearing pads made me wonder. Perhaps my urinary system was compromised by age or some undiagnosed problem. If I chose surgery, would a pre-existing issue make me need pads forever? Did I want that? While I didn't know what would happen after surgery, I didn't want to put myself in a situation to find out. This certainty bumped surgery from the number one slot to the number two slot, less than an hour after scheduling the operation.

What a roller coaster.

CHAPTER 10

Healing with Nature

THE NEXT DAY, I KNEW I NEEDED TIME AWAY FROM THE wilds of cancer. When I told Mary, she said she needed a break, too. We headed for some nature time in a national forest miles from Gardiner. We began our day hike strolling along a narrow path through a mix of tall, golden grasses that mesmerized us as they swayed in the breeze. When we entered the cool shade of a conifer-and-aspen forest, sunlight through the trees dappled the understory of colorful wildflowers. We strolled beside and crossed a creek several times. I tromped through the water without worrying about getting my boots wet. Mary stepped from rock to rock and kept hers dry.

As we followed this well-maintained trail through thick forest, we chatted about how we preferred hiking in Yellowstone's Northern Range, the part of the park closest to Gardiner. There, we avoided human trails and followed animal trails. Bison were our favorite trailblazers. We enjoyed moving through a vast, open landscape

dotted with sage, grasses, pines, and junipers. We marveled at the abundant views of mountains, valleys, and
plateaus. We'd had no such views so far.

At the hike's midpoint, we crossed another creek
and started climbing. The trail switchbacked to a sunlit
ridge, where we were finally rewarded with a view of
rugged mountain peaks in the Absaroka Range. The full
sun fed large patches of yellow, purple, and blue wildflowers beside us. We stopped and stood and savored
this combination of distant views and nearby beauty. I
could feel my emotional struggles of the last few days
dwindling—nature's healing. Just what I needed.

Though I had sought a day off, I couldn't help but notice
parallels between the hike and my cancer journey. Earlier
in the hike, although I had felt confined in the dense forest, I had enjoyed the beauty of the wildflowers and been
soothed by the sounds of the creek. Early in my journey
into the emotional darkness of the wilds of cancer, I had
enjoyed and been soothed by the support of Mary and
others. That support shone through like the sunbeams
that had dappled and nurtured this forest's understory.

Crossing creeks and getting my feet wet several times
reminded me of crossings made so far in my cancer journey.
One was when I learned that if prostate cancer spreads,
there is no likely cure yet. That crossing brought on tears,
but like my wet boots drying as we stood in the afternoon
sun, those tears and emotional discomfort faded over time.

As I stood on that ridgetop enjoying the view of distant mountains and trailside wildflowers, I felt myself

moving out of the present struggles and into an enticing picture of the future. I saw myself making a decision that ended this struggle to choose between surgery and radiation. Once I completed treatment, regardless of the outcome, I would maintain a life-affirming focus, enjoying the beauty in my life close at hand, delighting in distant views of my future, and spending healing time in wide-open and restorative countryside like that ridge.

I was not alone in feeling healed by time in nature. An article published by the *Yale School of the Environment* reports that a European study of 20,000 people found that those "who spent two hours a week in green spaces— local parks or other natural environments, either all at once or spaced over several visits—were substantially more likely to report good health and psychological well-being than those who don't."

The article quotes Richard Louv, who coined the term Nature Deficit Disorder and wrote one of the first books on the healing power of nature. He said that the academic world virtually ignored nature's healing power when he was writing his book in 2005. "I could find 60 studies that were good studies. Now it's approaching and about to pass 1,000 studies, and they point in one direction: Nature is not only nice to have, but it's a have-to-have for physical health and cognitive functioning."

Research indicates that spending time in nature provides distinct benefits. It can reduce anxiety, blood pressure, stress hormone levels, and nervous system arousal. It can improve immune system function, self-esteem, and mood. A study published by The National Library of Medicine found that the positive effects of nature on physical health, mental health, and social well-being "can increase with the dose of nature." The more, the merrier.

Researchers have offered several theories regarding nature's healing power, according to an article by the American Psychological Association. One theory proposes that "since our ancestors evolved in wild settings and relied on the environment for survival, we have an innate drive to connect with nature." Another suggests that time in nature triggers a physiological response that reduces stress levels. A third submits that being in nature restores our ability to concentrate and pay attention.

The APA article reports that trekking to remote locations adds value to the healing. A survey of more than 4,000 U.K. residents found that "people reported more connection to nature and felt more restored after visiting rural and coastal locations than they did after spending time in urban green spaces." Areas such as nature reserves and protected habitats were more beneficial than areas with less biodiversity.

Mladen Golubic, medical director of the Osher Center for Integrative Health, summarizes the healing power of nature this way: "Prioritizing your wellness by spending time in nature promotes physical activity, engages your senses, encourages social interaction, and enhances well-being—all key elements of keeping you healthy."

Clearly, spending time on that ridge in that national forest, in Yellowstone, and in our backyard was—and would continue to be—curative in my battle with cancer.

CHAPTER 11

A Plan

THE NEXT MORNING, I WAS BUSY IN OUR BACKYARD WATER-ing all those trees and shrubs we had planted to attract and nurture birds, bees, and butterflies. There was no question that our golden elderberry and chokeberry were nurturing. I sat and watched as a flock of starlings zoomed in, ate, and zoomed away again, again, and again.

After the restorative ridge and a morning among our winged and green friends, I felt rejuvenated and ready for another round of facing cancer and maybe even deciding on a treatment approach. I was thankful for nature's healing and glad to begin understanding the science behind it.

I left the yard, went inside, and found Mary. She said she had just watched videos from the Prostate Cancer Research Institute and learned about a relatively new scan, the PSMA PET. The doctor in one of the videos said that the PSMA PET made a nuclear bone scan — like the one I'd had — seem crude. Mary had also read a journal article predicting that in the future, doctors will start with a PSMA PET when assessing high-risk prostate cancer, like I have. Curious, we wanted to learn more and agreed to watch videos together.

Just a month after diagnosis, we had developed a research process that was simple but time-consuming. We aimed to gather the best information to make the best decisions. When we found a video or article from a reputable source with potentially useful information, we sought to confirm that information from at least a second reputable source, such as a scientific journal, a university specializing in cancer research, or an organization like the Prostate Cancer Foundation. Our efforts were ongoing; new research and technologies changed treatment approaches and outcomes.

When we found a Mayo Clinic video confirming the PSMA PET information, Mary stopped the video and said, "I feel like a weight has been lifted."

"What do you mean?"

"This new info gives us options. If you can get that scan, we'll have what we need to make the best treatment decisions."

"Yeah, I'm sure struggling. Just look at how the other day, I scheduled surgery, and an hour later, after talking to that man about his prostate cancer and incontinence, I was convinced that radiation would be a better choice."

Mary smiled and said, "If you want, I'll call the facility in Seattle and see if we can make an appointment for a PSMA scan there."

Her unwavering support moved me to tears. A few moments later, I was able to speak and said, "That would be so nice."

Mary's smile widened as she said, "I was going to do it anyway and not tell you till afterward."

Stress-relieving laughter filled the room.

We closed our business meeting with a plan. We would focus on radiation as the number one treatment option. That afternoon, during our first consultation with the oncologist, we would ask if he used PSMA PET scans. If he did, we would request one and continue working with him. If he didn't, we would look for a different oncologist. If we believed in the value of the PSMA PET, we needed a doctor who shared that belief.

CHAPTER 12

Decision Made

As we sat in the local cancer center awaiting that appointment with the oncologist, I watched the young man at the front desk interact with patients. He smiled for all, used the names of most, and laughed with many. The aide who took us to the exam room introduced herself and was friendly as she took my vitals. The next team member, a nurse, was pleasant as she educated us about radiation. After she left, the oncologist arrived. He was cordial, but also a "let's get down to business" kind of guy.

Before we began, I asked if I could record our conversation, and he approved. He said that based on my PSA and biopsy, my cancer fell into the very-high-risk category. I asked what that meant, and he explained that if radiation couldn't kill my cancer cells, they could become a life-threatening problem.

Ugh! Life-threatening. That's what the urologist said at our last appointment.

The oncologist went on to recommend a five-day-a-week radiation plan with forty-four treatments. When I asked about side effects, he explained that the edges of my bladder and rectum near the prostate would get irradiated and irritated. He would use a foam gel as a spacer between my rectum and prostate to protect my rectum. But as we moved into the third week of radiation, I might experience looser bowels and frequent urination with some burning. A month or so after treatment ended, I should be returning to normal. He added that most men were happy with their bowel and bladder functioning in the long term after radiation.

Because of my high-risk cancer, he also recommended hormone therapy for eighteen months. I'd be injected every four months with a medication that would stop my body's production of testosterone. That, in turn, would starve my testosterone-gobbling prostate cancer cells.

During hormone therapy, I would experience erectile dysfunction and lose interest in sex. Mary and I had read about those side effects and were concerned they would ruin our sex life. Of course, my dying from prostate cancer would have an even greater impact. I would also experience fatigue and hot flashes. The longer the therapy continued, I might lose bone density and muscle mass.

When I shared my doubts about agreeing to hormone therapy because of those side effects, the oncologist said that once treatment ended, "these biochemical changes should reverse." He strongly recommended I have the first injection, and when it came time for the next, we could decide whether to continue.

As I nodded in agreement, Mary asked about the possibility of a recurrence. He said a recurrence would most likely occur outside the prostate.

Oh, no, that's deadly, I thought. I asked for the odds.

He said, "About fifty-fifty."

As I sat silently, troubled by that coin-flip chance of a deadly recurrence, I sensed the consult would end soon, and I still had to ask about his experience. I felt as uncomfortable asking him as I had when I asked my urologist. I took a deep breath and asked, "How long have you been doing this?"

He rocked back in his chair, crossed his arms over his chest, and said, "A long time."

While his body language said the question bothered him, his answer didn't satisfy. I needed more. "Like how long?"

He blinked, stared, and said, "Twenty-five years, and this is the most common cancer I treat."

Satisfied, I prepared for the next big question: What was his opinion of the PSMA PET scan? I took another deep breath and asked. Without hesitation, he said it was a great scan and supported my desire to have one. I was relieved.

His description of hormone therapy, radiation treatment, and the side effects of both was similar to what Mary and I had found in our research. Impressed with his answers to questions and his chairside manner, I felt more confident about making radiation my first option and having him treat me. We had met our second guide on this journey.

CHAPTER 13

Sanctuary

LATER THAT AFTERNOON, WHEN MARY AND I ARRIVED HOME from the consult, we busied ourselves with yard work in relief-filled silence. She trimmed and watered shrubs. I collected fallen apples that might attract a local grizzly bear, busily building body fat before a long winter's sleep. Then, I headed inside for some sleep of my own; the consult and the fear of and uncertainty about prostate cancer treatment and its side effects had worn me out again.

After my nap, I sat at the computer and began transcribing the recording of the oncologist consult. I keyboarded about the five-day-a-week radiation plan, the forty-four treatments, the side effects, and the chance of a deadly recurrence. Though there was more to transcribe, I couldn't continue. I'd had enough of revisiting the consult and wondering what I could, should, or would be doing to my body, mind, and heart for the foreseeable future.

Instead, I dug into a digital file on how to care for our grass, shrubs, and trees. As I read and looked at photos,

I smiled and felt more confident that this drive to keep our green friends healthy—as shown with the ailing pine a couple of weeks ago—was somehow related to my drive to keep myself healthy.

I looked out the window; the backyard called. I gave the computer its nap, walked outside, slipped out of my shoes, and climbed into our hammock, which nestled under two shade trees. As I settled in, a mountain bluebird landed six feet from me, looked me in the eye, and offered a short, sweet song. The joy of that moment filled my heart and eased my mind. I thanked him for his kindness. Nature at work again.

While our quarter-acre yard looked and felt, as one friend had remarked, like a sanctuary, it was far from that when we bought the place. Then, the property was surrounded by a low wire fence that elk could jump over, and a bison had walked through, leaving a gaping hole. Since our four-legged neighbors could easily enter the yard to feast on any tasty fare we grew, we removed the useless fence and installed a taller wooden one. With our territory protected, we went to work. We huffed and puffed and changed the landscape by planting fifty or so trees and shrubs we nurtured to maturity.

Now, I had to commit to changing the landscape on which I would fight cancer. As we had replaced that old fence with a new one that kept grazers away, I would have to learn ways to keep cancer cells at bay. As Mary and I had researched which plants would make our yard a haven for bees, birds, and butterflies, we would research which habits would make my body a haven for healthy cells and a hostile environment for cancer cells.

I put my hands behind my head and stared at the leaves rustling in the breeze above the hammock. I closed my eyes and flashed back to some moments after that day's consult had ended. The oncologist wanted another blood sample. Since no staff were immediately available, Mary and I walked to an empty atrium to wait. I paced, rubbing my feet against the rough carpet, making a scratchy sound that mimicked my feelings.

Mary watched me and said, "You'll survive this, Rick. But you'll be dealing with it the rest of your life."

While my head agreed, my heart begged to differ: I feared I would not survive.

Looking around for any distraction, I spotted a gray plaque on the red brick wall. I shuffled over and read a quote from Eleanor Roosevelt: "You gain strength, courage, and confidence by every experience in which you really stop to look fear in the face... do the thing you think you cannot do."

I stepped back and let the words fade out of focus in my vision and into focus in my heart. My spirits lifted.

Wanting more, I scanned the atrium walls and found a plaque from Cayla Mills: "You never know how strong you are until being strong is the only choice you have."

As I savored the quotes, a nurse arrived and said it was time for a blood sample. After the blood work, Mary offered to drive us home. I was glad; I wouldn't have been an attentive driver. I was way too preoccupied with the quotes, the consult, and that coin-flip chance of recurrence.

I opened my eyes, swung out of the hammock, took a deep breath, and dug my toes into the soft grass. I felt relieved by that short nature break on such a trying day. Mary and I agreed that we had found the right place, team, and treatment to battle my cancer. Hormone therapy would begin in two weeks, radiation in five. While reacting to side effects that would hit me physically, mentally, and emotionally, I would have to devise ways to be proactive and help my body, mind, and heart be healthier and stronger on this daunting journey.

I did not know — could not know — the outcome, but I was willing to begin. I was ready, to paraphrase Eleanor Roosevelt, to stop and look fear in the face and do the thing I think I cannot do.

And I had this sanctuary to escape to when needed.

CHAPTER 14

Sugar, Sugar, Sugar

As we moved away from the struggle of choosing a treatment and toward the months of dealing with side effects from radiation and hormone therapy, Mary and I began exploring what we ate and drank. We started with something near and dear to our hearts: coffee. Each of us went online to research the relationship between coffee and prostate cancer. When Mary found conflicting information—coffee could help and coffee could harm—we agreed to dig deeper. I wanted findings that would keep coffee in my life.

The National Institutes of Health linked to a recent study that found "no evidence to support harmful effects of coffee consumption on prostate cancer risk." At the National Library of Medicine, another recent study concluded, "Higher coffee consumption was significantly associated with a lower risk of prostate cancer." That sounded good, but I couldn't help wondering how I, a three-to-four-cup-a-day guy, ended up with prostate cancer. Continuing to research, I was eventually satisfied that studies from reputable sources didn't call coffee conducive to prostate cancer.

I pushed away from the computer and headed to the kitchen to fix my second cup. But as I started to dump in a rounded tablespoon of sugar, I stopped and wondered about another relationship: sugar to prostate cancer. Fearing the worst, I returned the sugar to the bowl and headed back to the office, unsweetened coffee in hand, a frown on my face.

Back online, I sipped my coffee, winced at its bitterness, and moused around, seeking information that might keep sugar in my coffee and my life. If only I could be so lucky. I found a study in the *British Journal of Nutrition* stating: "Increased consumption of sugars from sugar-sweetened beverages was associated with increased risk of prostate cancer for men in the highest quartile of sugar consumption." I leaned back in my chair and shook my head; I was undoubtedly in that highest quartile, probably right at the top.

I had been a sugar addict all my adult life. Not only did I slug sugar-rich drinks, but I also added sugar to meals I cooked. I devoured processed foods with no regard for their added sugar. I ravaged sugar-filled desserts. I gobbled sugary candy while watching TV. Thankfully, I must have a high metabolism, because all that sugar hasn't made me overweight. But it might have helped bring on cancer.

Thinking about my sugary past, I wished I could turn back the clock. But that was behind me. All that was left was that day and the future. Feeling guilt and regret, I decided it was time for a nature break. I headed for the backyard.

Outside, I stood, closed my eyes, and turned toward the sun. I felt my face warm and my body relax. Tuning in to the buzz of bees, I opened my eyes, walked to a nearby flower pot, dropped to all fours, and watched a bee work. She went from flower to flower, never staying long. As she stepped across a blossom, she fed on the sugar-rich nectar that gave her the energy to be as busy as a bee. She also collected pollen particles, which she moistened and stuck to her hind legs. Eventually, she would buzz home with that sugar-rich pollen that would be turned into food to nourish her colony. She and her colony benefited from the sugar. No one benefited from my sugar habit. I was simply feeding my sweet tooth and sugar addiction.

I wanted to better understand the relationship between sugar and prostate cancer. I left the bee to her work and returned to mine. I discovered a recent article from the Prostate Cancer Foundation that stated: "Changing the diet—to one low in sugar, but also low in other carbohydrates which cause blood sugar to spike—can make cancer-fighting treatments work even better." Another PCF article advised against eating processed foods laced with added sugar. "Limit or eliminate refined sugar. Cancer loves sugar. You hate cancer. Do the math: next time you have a craving, grab a piece of fruit instead."

OK, OK, sugar had to go! Not just in my coffee but also in my diet. Damn! Disappointed yet determined, I pushed back from the computer, stomped to the garage, grabbed a big empty box, pounded to the pantry, and filled the box with products I had enjoyed but must now reject: sugary soft drinks (eight to ten teaspoons of sugar per twelve-ounce can), various kinds of candy (ten teaspoons of sugar in a half-cup serving of my favorite chocolate covered raisins), and even some staples, like ketchup (twenty-five percent sugar).

I grunted as I hefted the box onto the kitchen counter. Shocked by its weight, I wondered what to do next. While the bee would use the sugar she collected to feed her colony, what could I do with this box I had jammed full of sugar rejects? I laughed when I pictured placing the box in front of a friend and saying, "Here's stuff that might help you end up with cancer. Want some?" If I didn't go that route, food banks could use some of the items that were actually food. One way or another, these sugary products were out of our house and out of my life. So was adding sugar to my coffee and cooking.

Having begun to explore ways to fight cancer through diet, I was curious about other strategies we could use to take a proactive approach. What else could I do while my body was exposed to testosterone-lowering medication and cancer-targeting radiation?

But that was a question for another day. Work was finished; it was time to head back outside for another nature break. Hopefully, I could watch the bees work.

CHAPTER 15

Miles of Talking

A COUPLE OF DAYS LATER, I SAT ON A SOFA, ALTERNATING between journaling and gazing out the window of our seventh-floor hotel room, which overlooked Seattle's Lake Union. The lake was dark blue and cluttered with all sorts of watercraft: SUPs, kayaks, small motorboats, bigger sailboats, oversized yachts, and the occasional landing or leaving seaplane. The sky was a lighter blue and cloud-free, allowing the western sun to pour through the window.

An hour earlier, Mary and I had walked along the overdeveloped lakeshore, which was crammed with heat-absorbing sidewalks, roads, parking lots, and buildings. We became overheated and eager to return to the room, where the air conditioner did an excellent job of cooling us during Seattle's unusual heat wave.

We had arrived at the hotel after twelve hours of driving and talking through 700 miles and one time zone. Now, almost five weeks post-diagnosis, we had traveled from Montana so that I could have that much-touted PSMA PET scan at a Seattle facility.

Well before sunrise, when we exited our garage, we had Mary-made breakfast sandwiches and Rick-made lattes—sugar no longer added, of course—to enjoy as I took the first shift on our drive west. After the sandwiches calmed our bellies and the caffeine excited our brains, Mary said, "While we're going to be in the car all day, how about I tell you what I've learned about foods that fight cancer?"

"Sounds good to me."

I trusted Mary's approach to research; she had learned the hard way. Diagnosed with breast cancer thirty years ago, she did hours upon hours of research—most required sitting and sifting through paper journals at the public library. She persisted and educated herself. She declined to allow chemo and radiation into her body. Instead, she changed her diet, increased her exercise, and had a double mastectomy. I was grateful to have this cancer survivor—who I lovingly call an environmental paranoid—lead the way in diet research.

Mary opened her phone and read from her notes about foods we should eat or avoid. First on her list was eliminating refined and added sugar. I was glad to tell her I had begun that process. She described other changes: replace cow's milk with soy milk. Eliminate poultry, red meat, and animal-based cheeses. Reduce our intake of processed foods and increase our consumption of sea-food that helps fight cancer, such as canned mackerel, sardines, and tuna. Consume more cruciferous vegetables and salads enhanced with nuts, seeds, and beans. Make fresh fruit our evening treat while watching TV. When she finished her list, we digested these changes in silence.

A few miles later, I pulled into a rest area so we could switch drivers. Back on the highway, as the interstate climbed toward Lookout Pass, the Idaho border, and the Pacific Time Zone, I described to Mary my number crunching to calculate how many teaspoons of sugar this sugar addict consumed on an average workday years ago, before we were a couple.

Back then, I started my daily addiction with a cup of coffee with three teaspoons of sugar. I drank it while eating oatmeal topped with two teaspoons of sugar. On the way to work, I stopped at my favorite coffee shop for a coffee laden with sugar and chocolate, accompanied by a scone with sugary icing and sugar baked in. As the day wore on and my caffeine rush wore off, I drank a can of sweet soda while snacking on a pack of sugar-dusted mini-donuts. When the workday ended, I drove home for dinner, followed, of course, by dessert, such as a couple of scoops of sugar-rich ice cream.

With much embarrassment, I admitted that between breakfast and bed, I had consumed more than three times the current American Heart Association's sugar recommendation for men! As we crested the pass and descended toward Lake Coeur d'Alene, I revealed my guilt-laden thoughts on how that sugar addiction may have nurtured my prostate cancer cells.

Mary glanced at me and said, "Don't get down on yourself about that."

I stared out the window at a seemingly endless conifer forest and said, "I know getting down on myself doesn't make sense. There's nothing I can do about the past." I turned and looked at her, "But I want you to know how I feel."

"I'm glad you're sharing your feelings. But you know," she said with a knowing smile, "if diet can feed cancer, diet can fight cancer."

"I like the sound of that," I said, reaching over to hold her hand. "Let's fight it!" I yelled as I pumped my other hand, formed into a fist, into the air.

As we cruised across the Idaho panhandle, we discussed how adopting a cancer-fighting diet might affect us. We would need to change our shopping habits and start studying nutrition labels to avoid cancer feeders and find cancer fighters. Once we changed our diet, we might experience gastrointestinal issues as we transitioned from a meat-based, low-fiber diet to a plant-based, high-fiber diet. We might lose weight. Surely, I would without all that calorie-heavy sugar.

By the time we had talked away 650 miles and crested Washington's Snoqualmie Pass, we started to feel the press of Seattle. Our chatting centered on traffic and the distance to the hotel.

As I sat and savored the sun pouring through the Seattle hotel's window, I felt good that we were embarking on a long and proactive process of designing our cancer-fighting diet. That was something I could sink my teeth into.

CHAPTER 16

Fearing Side Effects

THE PSMA PET SCAN WAS COMPLETED, AND WE HAD returned home from Seattle. I was sitting on the deck, journal in my lap, feeling both physically and emotionally exhausted. As I put pen to paper, I remembered how, weeks earlier, I had declared that fighting cancer would be my full-time job. I was naive and had no idea just how all-consuming this battle would become.

For example, obtaining that fifteen-minute scan took four full days, partly due to a mix-up at the Seattle facility. When we arrived, I asked the receptionist to confirm that I was scheduled for a PSMA PET. She studied the computer for a long time and finally acknowledged that I was booked for a scan, but she couldn't confirm the type.

In the exam room. I asked a technician the same question. She studied the paperwork, shook her head, and said I was scheduled for a different scan, one that wouldn't be helpful. She left to call my Cancer Center and confirm which test they had ordered. When she returned, she apologized and said they had ordered a PSMA PET, but that somewhere along the line the order had been botched.

I asked if I could still have the procedure that day. She said I couldn't; the scan required some preparation that hadn't been done. Frustration building, I asked when I could have the scan. She didn't know. My frustration burst forth as I declared that I had driven from Montana, this trip was expensive, and I wasn't interested in leaving without the scan. She retreated to discuss rescheduling with other staff.

An hour later, she finally returned with good news: they could do the scan the next day. I confirmed it would be a PSMA PET and headed to the waiting area to find Mary and vent my frustration. The scan finally occurred, but it was so late that we decided to spend another night in Seattle rather than drive home in the dark.

As I journaled, I saw that frustrating and time-consuming experience as a lesson. Just like medical staff ask for my name and birthdate at each step from check-in to treatment, I must ask staff to confirm each treatment I'm about to receive.

I dropped my pen onto the journal and sat back, ready to watch the sprinkler heads in the yard go round and round, releasing a spray that I hoped would revive the lawn after a stretch of scorching July days.

As our grass had to handle the heat, I had to contend with cancer. I sighed and whispered to the yard, "I don't feel up to this fight." The thought entered my mind that

I could give up, stop fighting, and let cancer take me as the doctors predicted it would. Though I immediately rejected that scary idea, I had to pick up the pen and record it. I had to own that deadly notion. Had to get it out of me and onto paper.

Next, I wrote about a deep determination to not give up. I would fight, fight, fight! I would do everything I could to keep my body as healthy as possible for as long as possible.

Then, with sad acceptance, I jotted that I'm in this fight for the rest of my life; I'll live with the threat of recurrence after treatment ends.

While writing about giving up, fighting, and accepting pained me, I also felt relieved. That's what makes my journaling a much-needed visit to a paper therapist.

I closed the journal, wished the lawn luck, and headed to my office to go online and see if the PSMA PET results were available. I clicked around, found the report, took a deep breath, and read. The cancer was not in my lymph nodes! Not in my bones! Not anywhere distant from the prostate! I banged the desktop with my fist and shouted for joy.

I leaped out of the chair and rushed to tell Mary. She was still in bed, enjoying the coffee I had brought her that morning, as I do every morning. As I stood beside the bed and shared the news, she grinned and applauded. I burst into tears and climbed onto the bed. We snuggled and sobbed — tears of relief, tears of joy. We knew what we were fighting and where it did and didn't live.

The next milestone in this fight would soon be reached. In a couple of days, I would begin hormone therapy. After hours of researching that treatment, I had agreed to have the first of four possible injections. However, I wasn't eager to experience the side effects, especially the erectile dysfunction and loss of interest in sex created by the low testosterone levels induced by therapy. Mary and I knew that our sex life would suffer or vanish.

A few nights ago, after our last lovemaking, we had cuddled beneath the sheet. As I told Mary how I had always enjoyed our sex, I felt as if I was offering a eulogy at a memorial service. Recalling love for a now-gone friend. Describing moments of joy. Sharing feelings of loss.

Mary listened and then said, "Let's not say goodbye to sex yet." We laughed and held each other tightly.

As I thought about that intimate moment, the vision of a roller coaster appeared again. We were at the top, ready to begin the scary descent into the depths of treatment. Hopefully, after descending, we would climb again—however slowly—to another high point. And stay there for as long as we could as we aged toward an end that was much nearer than I would prefer, with or without cancer.

CHAPTER 17

Treatment Begins

AFTER THOSE EMOTIONALLY INTENSE DAYS AND BEFORE the soon-to-start hormone therapy, I needed to get out of my mind and heart and into my body and nature. I planned to spend a few hours being physical. As I mowed the lawn, ignoring the self-propelled feature and pushing the mower in full sun and 92-degree heat, the exertion and the sweat dripping down my face drove the stress away. When I finished mowing, I still wasn't ready to stop. I stood in the middle of the yard, looked around, and wondered what to do next. I spotted a few shrubs that could use trimming. I grabbed the hedge trimmer, walked to the bushes, and got busy.

Humming as I worked, my body, heart, and mind opened to memories of Lois, Mary's older sister. She had died eight years earlier from brain cancer. Mary and I were part of what Lois had called her A-Team. We took turns with two other pairs of family members caring for her. During her last year, as her condition deteriorated and her treatment intensified, we made the cross-country drive from Oregon to Maryland several times and lived with her for up to two months at a time. One stay was during a full-blown spring in Lois's big yard. Even while battling cancer, she spent time in that yard, weeding, mowing the lawn, and trimming shrubs. She wanted to beautify this home, her sanctuary, which she loved so much and did not want to leave.

As the hedge trimmer vibrated in my hands and the shrubs took shape, it made sense that I shared a heartfelt moment with Lois—a person I love and miss, a person who modeled how to battle cancer. I wished she were there to help me, not just with the yardwork, but also with the battle. She would have done both well. I hoped that my memories of her strength would help me handle hormone therapy and radiation.

The next day, Mary and I sat silently in the exam room until the oncologist tapped on the door and entered, pulling up his COVID-required mask. We exchanged greetings as he sat at the desk, positioned the keyboard, typed, and announced that he was pulling up images from my PSMA PET. I didn't tell him about the frustration and the four days spent on that scan. Instead, I stood and stared over his shoulder at the screen. He placed a forefinger just above a spot on a black-and-white image. He said the scan showed most of the cancer was right there, on the upper part of the prostate adjacent to the bladder.

He studied the image in silence and surprised me when he said that he was not going to recommend the foam gel he had earlier said he would use to put space between the prostate and the rectum. He was concerned that inserting the gel might block the radiation from hitting all the cancer cells; those not killed by radiation could spread.

"Does not using the gel mean more possibility of damage to my rectum?" I asked.

He shook his head emphatically. "I treated patients for twenty-two years without hydrogel and rarely had any long-term rectal issues."

He studied the image again and said that even though the PSMA PET showed no cancer in the lymph nodes, "Statistically, there's a pretty good chance that there are some microscopic deposits." He recommended radiating the lymph nodes near the prostate.

As I wondered if I had again been naive when I told Mary the great news from the PSMA PET report, and we had cried with relief, he turned to me and asked, "So what are the side effects of the hormone therapy?"

"You're asking me?"

He nodded.

I replied like a pupil to a teacher: "Erectile dysfunction, loss of sex drive, hot flashes. Some men experience brain fog."

When he nodded approval, the high achiever within me took a bow. Then he said, "You got most of them. There's also loss of muscle mass and bone density when hormone therapy goes on for a long time."

As he turned to the screen and tapped a few more keys, I recalled that eighteen months of hormone therapy qualified as a long time. "Yeah, I read about that. And I plan to fight those losses with diet and exercise, things I can control." He turned toward me and appeared interested, so I continued. "I'm committed to exercising, running, biking, hiking, cross-country skiing, and strength and stretch workouts. Do you have any concerns about that?"

Lines from a mask-hidden smile formed at the corner of his eyes as he shook his head from side to side. "I wish more of my patients did that."

As my inner high achiever glowed and took another bow, Mary asked, "How soon is the onset of side effects?" The glow dimmed.

"At a biochemical level, within the first couple weeks, we're going to start seeing these changes." But, he added, any measurable change in bone density would take at least a year, and my being active would help reduce the loss of bone density and muscle mass.

He turned to the computer, hit several keys, and the screen went dark. I assumed this meant our time was up and thanked him for answering our questions. He stood, headed for the door, and said he would have the nurse prepare the injection.

A short while later, the nurse entered the room, needle in hand. After we chatted for a moment, I asked if that needle contained the first hormone therapy injection. She glanced at the needle and then at me, seemed surprised that I had asked, but confirmed that it was. Mary described the recent mix-up in Seattle with the PSMA PET scan, which prompted us to double-check everything.

The nurse stared intently over her mask, pointed a finger at us, and exclaimed, "That's good! You definitely should." She explained that since the pandemic began, healthcare workers have been overwhelmed. Mistakes have been made and will continue to be made. It's up to us—the patients—to double-check and help avoid mistakes, she said.

We thanked her for that affirmation. She nodded, the shot went in without pain, and six weeks after diagnosis, the next leg of my journey officially began. I would soon discover how I would handle treatment and side effects.

CHAPTER 18

DARE to Fight Cancer

DURING THE WEEKS WE STRUGGLED TO DECIDE WHICH medical provider and treatment to choose, Mary and I often asked ourselves, *What can we do to help? How can we be proactive rather than reactive?* In answering those questions, we identified four areas that we could control to help us and our medical team: diet, attitude, rest, and exercise. I created an acronym, DARE, to represent the four.

As I focused on exercise, the E, I purchased a fitness watch to help track my efforts and progress. I also bought new sweatpants. I put both on one night and did a fashion show for Mary. As I turned circles in front of her and grinned like a madman, she giggled and cooed, "You have such a svelte body." When I flexed my skimpy arm muscles for her viewing pleasure, we both burst out laughing.

As the laughter died, I turned to Mary and, holding out my arm adorned with that new watch, asked her in a lousy Clint Eastwood imitation, "Hey, beautiful, you want to know what time it is?" She laughed, rolled her eyes, waved me away, and muttered, "No, thanks."

I couldn't help myself. At seventy-three, I was eager to delve deeper into exercise. For the last couple of years, I had watched my old sweatpants deteriorate. I hadn't considered replacing them since I rarely ran or biked anymore. Instead, I spent more time hiking and cross-country skiing, which required different clothing.

We love cross-country skiing. One winter, before diagnosis, we skied on forty different days, often with friends. But as treatment progressed and side effects increased in the coming winter, I feared I would not feel up to skiing as much. I would miss the crunch of the skis as I took my turn breaking trail in deep, fresh snow. I would miss the whisper of the skis as we delighted in a downhill reward for the climbing we sought and enjoyed. I would miss the contrast of sweat on my chest as clouds of my breath drifted away. I would miss the time bonding with friends in nature.

However, while I might ski less, research has convinced me that a variety of exercises is essential to a proactive approach to fighting my cancer. I would start slow and easy, not pushing for personal bests. For a man my age (There it is again!), this was not about striving for speed; this was about filling a need. I needed to get my aging body in the best shape possible, not just to fight but to beat cancer. I was glad the radiation oncologist had no concerns when I had described my exercise plans.

Mary continued researching, designing, and feeding us a plant-based diet, the D. She started preparing enjoyable new meals several weeks ago. I did not doubt that the diet would support my body during exercise. Our research indicated it would also cut off some essential nutrients for my cancer cells—especially sugar spikes. Great! The weaker they became, the happier I would be.

While cancer changed how I fed and exercised my body, it also invaded my dreams and rest, the R. One night, my dream-induced struggling and grunting roused Mary. Sliding close and wrapping her arms around me, she asked if I wanted to discuss the dream. I said I didn't recall many details, but I felt that this dream, like the one the night before, was cancer-inspired. In both dreams, some bad people were trying to capture me and take me to a place I didn't want to go. I fought them and kept yelling, "I'm not going to let you win!"

Whatever challenges I faced, asleep or awake, I was glad I had adopted an attitude, the A, of being ready and willing to fight. As supportive friends had reminded me, I needed to be myself. I needed to go deep into this journey into the wilds of cancer, just as I had always immersed myself in whatever interested me: Yellowstone, wildlife advocacy, bike touring, backcountry hiking, writing, photography, and now our approach to fighting—and hopefully beating—cancer.

While developing DARE, I heard a doctor mention Lifestyle Medicine in a webinar. Intrigued, I researched the topic. According to a journal article authored by eight

MDs and titled *Foundation of Lifestyle Medicine and Its Evolution*, this new medical specialty is one of the fastest-growing in America. It uses well-researched lifestyle changes to prevent, manage, and reverse chronic diseases.

Lifestyle Medicine has six pillars: a whole-food, plant-based diet; regular physical activity; restorative sleep; effective stress management; avoidance of risky substances; and positive social connections. I saw those pillars as consistent with our focus on diet, attitude, rest, and exercise.

The authors provide an example of the importance of exercise for health and longevity. In a study of over 4,800 individuals spanning ten years, the number of daily steps taken was significantly associated with decreased mortality, particularly among those aged sixty-five and older. The more steps, the better.

The authors also highlight the importance of sleep. Following Lifestyle Medicine guidelines results in sleep that helps the body repair and restore itself every night. Conversely, consistently poor sleep can lead to cognitive impairment, suppression of the immune system, cardiovascular disease, diabetes, hypertension, inflammation, anxiety, depression, and early death.

The article explains how high stress levels can cause serious harm. Stress may lead to inactivity, non-restorative sleep, and unhealthy food choices. Spending time in nature and using mind-body techniques, such as biofeedback, meditation, and mindful movement practices like yoga or tai chi, can help reduce stress.

Another study, this one by the American College of Lifestyle Medicine and published in the *Journal of Nutrition*, reviewed the clinical practice guidelines that provide dietary recommendations. Clinical practice guidelines are based on current medical knowledge and evidence. When clinicians follow the guidelines, they provide consistency in clinical care.

The researchers analyzed the guidelines published during a recent twelve-year period. In general, the guidelines promoted the consumption of vegetables, beans, lentils, peas, fruits, nuts, seeds, whole grains, and low-fat dairy products. They discouraged the consumption of alcohol, sodium, sweets, added sugar, and sweetened beverages. I was pleased to read that the diet we had developed was consistent with those guidelines.

The American College of Lifestyle Medicine offers certification to doctors and other health practitioners. The ACLM recently reported that in the first five years after it began certifying, more than 3,000 U.S. physicians and other health professionals had become certified in Lifestyle Medicine. Given that there are almost five million LPNs, RNs, nurse practitioners, physician assistants, medical assistants, and physicians in the U.S., that's a start, but not many certifications.

The doctors who wrote *Foundation of Lifestyle Medicine and Its Evolution* have thoughts about this certification delay. They note that physicians often exhibit poor lifestyle habits. This complicates the adoption of Lifestyle Medicine "because evidence shows that overweight, inactive, poorly nourished physicians who neglect self-care themselves are less likely to inquire about or provide effective guidance regarding these crucial lifestyle factors." They also point to limited awareness and education about Lifestyle Medicine among healthcare professionals, policymakers, and the general public.

While Lifestyle Medicine may not be widespread yet, Mary and I undoubtedly practiced it with DARE. The research convinced me that I needed to investigate both approaches even further to help keep my body, mind, and heart healthy while subjected to radiation and hormone therapy.

CHAPTER 19

Q&A

MARY AND I WERE TALKING OVER THE SPEAKERPHONE with a friend about cancer. When our friend asked how I handled the emotional side of this struggle, I explained that we deal with this disease and dilemma by exploring optimism and pessimism, voicing hopes and fears, and sharing tears and laughter.

I mentioned that I journal every day and occasionally have helpful phone and email conversations in which I share my journey with a few friends. I described how such sharing accomplishes several things. It decreases my fear of cancer and also lets others know what I'm battling. That creates the possibility of receiving much-needed support that can be part of the cure.

After the phone call ended, I wondered whether there was scientific evidence supporting the idea that maintaining a positive attitude, sharing feelings, and finding support help a person beat cancer. Time to go back online to discover what reputable sources had to say.

I settled onto the American Cancer Society website, where an article by the ACS medical and editorial content team answered four critical questions.

First was a question I had asked myself, especially during the bargaining phase of grieving: *Did I bring on cancer?*

The ACS answer: "Your personality and emotions did not cause your cancer. Research on this topic has not shown a link between personality and overall cancer risk."

The second question provided a different insight into maintaining a positive attitude: *Will a positive attitude improve my quality of life and chance of surviving cancer?*

The ACS answer: "People with cancer might hear from others that they should stay positive. But there is no right or wrong way to live with a cancer diagnosis, because it affects everyone differently. It's important to remember that feeling distress, depression, fear, or anxiety is normal when learning to deal with a serious illness such as cancer. It's also important to recognize and talk about these feelings with someone. Maybe this is a friend, family member, or clergy member. Many people find it helpful to join a support group or seek counseling."

Third was another relevant question: *Can support groups and counseling help me?*

The ACS answer: "Research has not shown that support groups or counseling help people with cancer live longer. However, there are many benefits for people with cancer who participate in support groups. Research shows that giving people with cancer information in a support group helps reduce tension, anxiety, and tiredness, and may lower the risk of depression. Sharing experiences with others can also improve feelings of well-being and overall quality of life."

The fourth question intrigued me: *Can I control the cancer by thinking myself well?*

The ACS answer: "Research has not shown that techniques like guided imagery, relaxation, or meditation can control cancer growth. However, these techniques can help manage some side effects and emotions related to cancer and cancer treatment. Pain, fatigue, nausea, vomiting, distress, anxiety, and depression can be helped with these and some other techniques. Managing these side effects and emotions may also improve quality of life."

Reading the Q&A strengthened my motivation to create a support system where I could honestly share with others what I faced and felt. A week after treatment began, I decided to build part of that system by connecting and reconnecting emotionally with a few men friends. I would also join a monthly, facilitated men's support group for prostate cancer patients offered by a local cancer-fighting organization.

I wanted my support system to help me maintain a positive attitude, reduce stress, and keep me motivated and focused on using DARE to give my body, mind, and heart what each needed to fight prostate cancer and treatment side effects.

CHAPTER 20

A Lakeside Moment

Two weeks after treatment began, Mary and I needed and took another break from the wilds of cancer. Early in the morning, we paddled our canoe at a small local lake and struggled to find a way through a green wall of rushes rising four to five feet above the lake's surface. When we reached an area with fewer rushes, we pushed gently into the thin, round stalks that gracefully bent to either side, hissed as they rubbed against the canoe, and allowed us entry into their extraordinary world.

Once through the gateway, we were happy to enter and follow a narrow channel to a small oval of open water. We stopped paddling, sat silently, and waited patiently for the residents of the rushes to accept our presence and resume their morning activities.

We soon heard birds fluttering among the stalks, but we couldn't find them. Mary did spot a partially concealed bird nest. About two feet above the water, the builders—perhaps marsh wrens or red-winged blackbirds—had woven dried rushes and grasses around several standing rushes and created a cone-shaped nest. Though we didn't see the builders, we heard some nearby birds emitting what sounded like alarm calls. We paddled quietly away and left them in peace.

We moved silently along another narrow channel until Mary caught sight of a painted turtle plodding across a mat of fallen golden vegetation. When the turtle craned its head to look back at us with its intent, tiny eyes, I grabbed my camera and zoomed in with the telephoto. I giggled when I spotted small blades of grass protruding from its mouth. As I clicked away, the turtle continued eating. While I was relieved that our presence was not changing its behavior, we knew we were intruding. We left the turtle to its meal and paddled on.

As we exited the world of the rushes and reentered the open lake, we were greeted by a wind strong enough to push our canoe to the side. We had to change our paddling to keep moving straight ahead. Yet we had not felt the wind while within the rushes. I marveled at how the birds knew to put their nests in such a protected area.

As we pointed the canoe across the lake and back to camp, a shadow crossed the water and our canoe. We looked up and spotted an osprey flapping toward the open part of the lake with a fish dangling from its claws. Wow! Behind and above the osprey flew a much larger bald eagle. Its white head and tail flashed in the morning sun. Wow! Wow! When the osprey banked to the right, so did the eagle. But no attack. As the osprey banked to the left, the fish slipped from its claws and splashed into the water. Surprisingly, neither fish-eater dove to retrieve the meal. The osprey veered right, the eagle left. The fish disappeared into the lake, probably happy to be home and alive, though a little banged up.

We paddled to camp, disembarked, and joined our friends lakeside. As afternoon slid into evening, I felt fully present and not burdened by cancer thoughts and worries as we enjoyed watching grebes, coots, and ruddy ducks interact on the open lake. Our visit was a success. Nature had healed again.

Once the sun set, Mary and I strolled to our little teardrop trailer parked under a massive, old cottonwood on the lakeshore. I smiled at the rough purring of a sandhill crane, imagining it was bidding us good night. In the middle of the night, as I tossed and turned with cancer worries that had snuck back in, an owl's hooting stilled me and lulled me back to sleep.

The next morning, I sat and journaled by the lakeside as redwing blackbirds, magpies, ducks, and a gathering of songbirds orchestrated a delightful wake-up concert. But nature's music did not dispel my need to visit my paper therapist. I grabbed my journal and pen and wrote about one of my cancer worries. Since diagnosis, I had been surprised to find myself showing Mary how to do specific household tasks that were usually mine. I hadn't told her why I was doing so. I hadn't confessed that I was trying to help her face what she called "life without

Rick." My unstated fear that cancer might take me was more significant than I was willing to admit.

Troubled by that scary thought, I put the pen down and gazed. Watching gentle green ripples flow across the lake calmed me. Beyond the lake, the morning light showcased a mountain range with peaks extending across the horizon. The sun warmed the right side of my face as a breeze cooled the left. Opposites at work. Healthy and sick. Present and absent. Life and death.

My heart was processing the possibility of losing my connection with family and friends, as well as this wonder-filled natural world that comforted me as I sat lakeside.

CHAPTER 21

Troubled Morning

A COUPLE OF DAYS LATER, I WAS SITTING ON THE DECK just before sunrise, again contemplating Electric Peak, struggling to recall a dream that—like others since my diagnosis—had filled me with foreboding. A veil of smoke from unseen and distant wildfires covered the peak. The gray layer and low morning light made the scene as ominous as the feelings within me.

Why was that morning the polar opposite of the previous day, when I had enjoyed a refreshing run on a favorite route along the Yellowstone River?

After jogging up and down two hills, I continued along a narrow gravel road that bisected a small ranch. Cattle grazed contentedly beside the road and behind a barbed wire fence. I glanced at my fitness watch and saw I was cruising at a decent aerobic pace. My inner high achiever thought, *Let's sprint and see if I can get my heart rate up further, maybe even to the max.* Instead, I put my hands in front of me, palms up and out, and disturbed the cattle by shouting, "Hold it, Rick, just enjoy what you're doing. The peace, the quiet, the fact you can still enjoy this at your age." I took my advice, cooed an apology to the cattle, and continued running at a reasonable pace. The cattle returned to feeding.

I ended the run stretching on an inviting little bridge that spans a narrow creek. I watched the water flow beneath me and felt the flow of run-generated joy within me.

Scientists once thought that the rush we feel from exercise came only from endorphins. But recent research reported in the *New York Times* reveals a "more complex cocktail of other key 'feel-good' chemicals produced during movement." The most potent of the neurochemicals in that cocktail is endocannabinoids, "which share a similar molecular structure with THC [a chemical compound found in cannabis], and bind to the same receptors in the brain—giving you that buzzy feeling that all is right in the world."

The article describes how "…it seems to take at least 20 minutes of moderate aerobic activity for the endocannabinoid system to kick in and start to lift your mood." And that holds true whether you're new to exercise or an elite athlete. "The longer you're able to sustain an aerobic workout at a moderate level of intensity—one in which you could carry on a conversation without becoming winded—the more your endocannabinoids will be flowing, and the higher your boost will be."

Standing on the bridge, grinning as endocannabinoids and endorphins fired and flowed, I was happy that exercising had become something I was proud of, not just another task checked off during a busy day when climbing a career ladder took precedence over caring for my body. Retired, I had time to take my time, battle for my body, and focus on my future. And I must. Exercise was more than a check box on my DARE to-do list. A variety of exercises had become crucial and enjoyable weapons in my battle against prostate cancer, along with diet, attitude, and rest.

Leaving the bridge, I went home and puttered around in the yard. I wanted to maintain that emotional high from the run. Occasionally, troubled feelings about cancer, treatment, and side effects tried to molest my mood. But I resisted and didn't dig into them. Instead, I dug into being in the yard. I climbed into bed that night, tired and happy after a day soothed by exercise and time in nature.

So why the troubled dream and the troubled morning after such a trouble-free day?

I uncovered one cause for concern as I visited my paper therapist and the rising sun warmed me on the deck. In a few days, I would return to the Cancer Center to have the team measure my body so they could plan how to radiate me. They would take a blood sample and test for my PSA level. I wanted the test to reveal that my PSA had decreased. That hormone therapy was already starving my cancer cells a month after the first injection. But I was scared it wouldn't.

Once radiation began, my body would be subjected to forty-four treatments. Five days a week for nine weeks, I would drive to the Cancer Center, climb onto the machine, and be radiated. Radiation side effects would hamper my daily activities and compound the hormone therapy side effects.

This side effects-filled descent into months and perhaps years of my body battling prostate cancer was what troubled me. As I closed my journal and returned to gazing at Electric Peak, I was glad my mind had deciphered what my heart was trying to tell me. I was indeed on a journey of body, mind, and heart.

CHAPTER 22

An Overarching Goal

ONE EVENING, A WEEK AFTER THE RADIATION PLANNING session and a week before the start of radiating my prostate, Mary and I sat on the sofa, watching TV. My attention was ripped from the show when I felt the burn of another hot flash, a significant side effect of the hormone therapy that began six weeks ago. The heat from this flash seemed more intense than usual. A light sweat formed and dripped down my neck and upper chest. I also felt a slight ache on the right side of my groin. Was that from exercising? I felt around down there while trying to keep Mary from noticing. Finally, I stood up, said not a word, and headed for the ibuprofen in its usual spot on the kitchen counter.

Mary heard the pills rattle in the bottle as I unscrewed the top. "Are you all right?" she asked, concern evident.

"I'm having a little groin pain," I said over my shoulder. "Probably just a cramping muscle. I'm working out regularly, so I'm bound to have aches and pains now and then. No big deal. Right?"

I tried to sound confident that this was a minor problem. But as I washed two ibuprofen down with a glass of water, I felt the opposite: I was scared, imagining that my body—my world—was falling apart. Would the hot flashes get worse? Would I injure myself by exercising too much and have to stop when I needed exercise the most? Would I devour too many ibuprofen and damage some organs?

Aargh! Cancer had taken over my life! I journaled every morning to maintain a cancer-fighting attitude. Then a cancer-fighting breakfast. Then cancer-fighting exercise. Then cancer-fighting research. Then a cancer-fighting lunch followed by a cancer-fighting nap.

Filling my days with fighting cancer had taken its toll. I no longer had the energy or interest to write my two Substack publications, *Love the Wild* and *Save the Wild*, about my love of and advocating for wildlife and wild lands. I hadn't posted a photograph or slideshow to social media in over a month. Writing, speaking, and photographing to protect wildlife and wild lands had been how I defined and presented myself to the world. But in the three months since diagnosis, I had morphed into an achy old guy who used to do that before he got cancer.

Though I no longer advocated, I found myself viewing cancer based on what I had learned while advocating for wolves and bison. To do what comes naturally—to sustain or increase their population—these wild critters need territory that provides room to reproduce and food for their pregnant bodies and young ones. But wolves in the West are kept from needed territory by being viewed as vermin or looters to be shot, poisoned, or trapped. Yellowstone's bison, natural migrators, are often hazed back into the park or shot as they leave because they are viewed as hungry intruders that compete with cattle for the same grazing grounds. Wolves and bison struggle to survive because of this conflict with us territory-hungry humans who claim wild lands and are unwilling to share.

Like wolves and bison, prostate cancer cells need food, such as testosterone and blood sugar spikes, to sustain or grow their population. Like wolves and bison, these tiny critters could disperse to find what they need. They could migrate from my radiated and wrecked prostate to better territory: my lymph nodes, liver, lungs, or bones. If they spread, a cure looked unlikely, though there is, as I write this, exciting research on emerging treatments to control and manage symptoms and pain for varying lengths of time after prostate cancer has spread.

The solution would be to make sure my cancer cells couldn't eat, reproduce, or migrate. Hormone therapy could starve them. Radiation could kill them. But that was treatment's job, not mine. Since I wasn't sure that radiation and hormone therapy would kill all the microscopic cells, my job would be to make sure that the tough little survivors did not find what they needed. I had to transform my body into an environment that would keep the wildlife inside me hungry, weak, and less likely to reproduce, spread, or survive.

Viewing my cancer cells as wildlife led me to finalize a long-term objective: I would make my body a hostile environment for prostate cancer cells and a haven for healthy cells. I would monitor my thoughts, feelings, and actions with that goal in mind. When I found myself drooling over some chocolate chip cookies, for example, I would remind myself that digesting the load of sugar in them would cause a blood sugar spike, creating a friendly environment for cancer cells. When I did not want to do my scheduled workout, I would remind myself that missing the workout would make my body less of a hostile environment for cancer cells. When I felt bored with our plant-based diet, I would remind myself that the diet made my body a haven for healthy cells and a hostile environment for cancer cells. Like it or not, I needed to organize every day around fighting cancer.

I put the ibuprofen bottle back on the counter, returned to the sofa, smiled at Mary, and hoped she didn't push me to talk. Thankfully, she obliged. But later, when we crawled into bed, she put her head on my chest—*Uh-oh, the talk position*—and asked, "Do you want to talk about what's going on?"

I didn't answer. Instead, I lay there, wondering if I wanted to talk. That was unusual since Mary and I had committed years ago to sharing our feelings, "saying the words," as we call it. Finally, I blurted, "I don't want to have prostate cancer."

"I don't want you to have it either, but you'll get through this. You're going to beat cancer."

"Sometimes, like tonight, it doesn't feel that way. I'm really scared about radiation starting and what all those shots are going to do to my body. I'm already struggling with the side effects of hormone therapy."

"That's understandable. You're entering the next phase of treatment, and we don't know how your body is going to react. But don't put on a smiley face when you're troubled. Please let me know what's going on. I want to be here to support you."

I felt that support and her body's warmth as we settled into silence. I began to relax as a tough day came to a close. I didn't know — couldn't know — what the future would bring. But I knew Mary would be there to support me. I also knew that I had that overarching goal to aspire to and keep me focused on fighting cancer every day. Some days would be painful. But reaching that goal every day could help keep me alive.

CHAPTER 23

Forest Bathing

AFTER THAT DAY OF WONDERING IF PROSTATE CANCER WAS wrecking my world, Mary and I realized it was time to seek refuge and relief in the natural world. With the morning sun just over the mountains, we began a hike, one of our favorites, to a collection of small lakes around Rainbow Lake. It was just the two of us, and that was intentional. We hadn't hiked without friends in quite some time. We looked forward to moving together, at our own pace, often in silence.

The hike took us up and down the rumpled hills below Sepulcher Mountain, another peak we can see from our dining room window. There was no formal trail; instead, we meandered along animal trails. We often stopped to delight in distant views or study something at our feet, such as when we stood among the white stems and yellow flowers of rabbitbrush, teeming with native bees. Captivated, I kneeled and, surrounded by buzzing and beauty, photographed the bees, a favorite subject.

When we arrived at the first of the lakes, we spotted three pronghorn farther up the rumpled hills. Once I pulled them into focus with the telephoto, I saw them staring at us with their incredible distance vision. I heard them snorting, perhaps communicating with one another—or telling us two-legged intruders to get lost. Moments later, they left, prancing upslope and behind some hills, seeking privacy. I turned my attention back to the lake. The surface was light brown, dotted with darker brown areas. Ducks paddled here and there, quacking and feeding.

We followed another animal trail up the rumpled hills toward two more lakes. I located one lake's rushing outlet stream, revealed by its gurgling but concealed by grasses and cattails. I followed the stream toward the lake, and as I came around a mound, some of the ducks on this lake spotted me and made a noisy departure. The rest, perhaps two dozen, gathered into a flock—security in numbers—and paddled across the blue surface toward a distant bank.

Mary and I meandered along the lake's edge toward a tall old conifer. We hopped across a noisy connector stream between this lake and its nearby neighbor. When we reached the conifer, we said hello, hugged its trunk, and settled down to relax and nestle alongside the thick, exposed roots of that big green friend we had visited many times.

That was our destination—a place to sit quietly and observe. Rabbitbrush and sage thrived in the cracked, dry soil around us. Looking across the lake and into the distance, we enjoyed a grand view of a canyon that the Yellowstone River had cut over thousands of years. A colorful slide graced one side of the canyon, rugged mountains formed the other.

Sheltered in the shade, we scanned and snacked in silence. I rubbed my back gently against the old tree's thick, rough bark, hoping to receive some of its strength and ability to survive so many challenges over so many years. I felt yesterday's fears falling away as I did my version of forest bathing.

Forest bathing, also known as shinrin-yoku in Japanese, is an established and studied Japanese medical practice that involves relaxing and connecting with nature in a forest setting. The intention is to be present in the moment and immerse yourself in the environment by engaging all your senses: sight, sound, smell, touch, and taste.

According to an article on the UC Berkeley website, more than a quarter of Japan's population participates in forest bathing. About one hundred officially sanctioned forest baths have guides to help users partake. The benefits of forest bathing continue for days after a visit.

The National Library of Medicine published an article by a Japanese researcher on a team that has established a new field of medical science called Forest Medicine, which studies the effects of forest bathing. Researchers have found that forest bathing increases the number and activity of natural killer cells, which destroy infected and diseased cells, including cancer cells. Forest bathing has been shown to improve sleep quality and reduce blood pressure, heart rate, and stress hormones. When tested, forest bathers exhibit increased vigor and decreased anxiety, depression, anger, fatigue, and confusion.

I was certainly feeling a reduction in cancer-related anxiety as I sat beneath and rubbed against our big green friend.

Beside me, Mary whispered, "We're incredibly lucky to live here."

"We sure are. I love this place and want to stay here forever—however long that is now that cancer has entered the picture."

We fell back into silence until we agreed to pack up and follow another animal trail toward another lake. Along the way, we discovered an area where tall golden grasses had been flattened to make soft sleeping spots, perhaps by the pronghorn who had made their noisy departure earlier.

When we reached the lake, we were stunned by its busy beauty. Along the bank, small patches of pink blossoms decorated the lake's surface. Thousands of dragonflies danced through the air just above the cattails and grasses everywhere we looked. Most were flying attached to each other in mating pairs. What was their function in that ecosystem? Why mate now, with cold and snow possibly just weeks away? Moments and questions like those made living here the learning experience we both enjoy.

Ready to end our forest bathing and head home, we climbed atop a mound, turned, and took one last look around. We each offered soft goodbyes to these lakes we hiked to every year, sometimes more than once.

As our words drifted away and silence returned, I whispered to the lakes, "I hope to see you next year."

"You will," said Mary, "You will."

I smiled and took her hand as we started sauntering back to the car. Once again, bathing in nature relieved, refreshed, and rejuvenated me.

CHAPTER 24

Drinking and Driving

I WAS DRIVING ALONE TO MY FOURTH RADIATION TREATMENT; Mary had an appointment elsewhere. To entertain myself for this thirty-minute trip, I set my phone to shuffle through its song library and play through the car's sound system. Then, I started chugging water to fill and swell my bladder, as instructed by my medical team. The swelling helped move some of the bladder away from the irradiated area and protect it. I dubbed this routine "drinking and driving," guzzling water, singing along to music, and enjoying the beautiful, colorful countryside as I drove to treatment.

Alongside the freeway, tall golden grasses waved in the breeze. The hills on both sides of the highway were flush with fall colors: dark green conifers and aspen in shades of green, yellow, and orange. Willows painted a small wetland red and yellow. The sky was a deep Montana blue. Mid-afternoon traffic was light, so I set the cruise control, adjusted my seat, and drove along under the influence of nature, water, and music.

I've been a singer for much of my adult life. Most of my singing has been with a steering wheel in my hands, eyes on the road, and joy in my heart. But I've also sung to audiences. I never earned a living performing, but I spent many joyful hours harmonizing with partners in a cappella groups that always included Mary. I loved the waves of applause that washed over us.

A memory of that applause snuck in when I finished singing along with a tune I used to sing lead on. I smiled as I recalled looking down into the front row of the audience at bright eyes, big smiles, and clapping hands. That memory filled me with joy—and a bit of sadness that those days were gone.

The following number was one I had sung along with on my way to the nuclear bone scan a couple of months ago. Then, I felt battered by this life-threatening disease and feared that my prostate cancer had spread. I had sung soulfully and cried. But as I sang along while driving to radiation treatment, I had that memory but no tears. I seemed to be over the initial shock and awe of the diagnosis. I knew that since my cancer had not yet spread, it was beatable. I felt optimistic.

I sang along with a few more favorites while gawking at the natural beauty I was drinking and driving through. Finally, I parked the car in the lot at the Cancer Center. A radiation table awaited. It was day four of forty-four. *Let's go, bladder buddy; You better be full.* I stepped out of the car and into the battle.

As I walked toward the Cancer Center, I was buoyed

by music and memories, lyrics and laughter, songs and sadness, heartache and harmony from miles of drinking and driving.

When I took a seat in the waiting room, I was wearing a gray t-shirt and the Center's loose-fitting blue scrubs. I was reading a novel on my phone about a man overcoming incredible odds — how appropriate — when another patient arrived and stood near the empty chair beside me. He was tall and dressed in worn jeans and a t-shirt that revealed well-muscled arms and a slight pot belly. He had a shaved head with wrap-around sunglasses perched on top. He looked like he had just come from work, a blue-collar job.

I made eye contact, smiled, and nodded a silent greeting. He nodded, sat in the chair, and started scrolling on his phone. As I returned to reading on mine, I felt a desire to begin conversing for the first time with another man who was here for cancer treatment. But I remained shy and silent until he put down his phone, pointed at my pants, and said, "Do I have to wear those scrubs in here?"

"I have to because I have prostate cancer." I started to show him the closet where the scrubs were stored when I realized that I didn't know anything about his cancer. "I think what you wear depends on where you're getting radiated." I touched my hand to my groin and said, "I'm getting radiated down here, so I wear these scrubs and no underwear. What kind of cancer do you have?"

"Brain," he said. I waited for more, but he didn't elaborate.

"Oh, brain, that's too bad." Unsure if his one-word response signaled I was intruding, I risked a question: "Is this your first treatment?"

"It is this time around."

"How many times have you been treated?"

"Two times with radiation and a couple of surgeries."

"Oh, this has been some ordeal, hasn't it?"

"Well," he said, "it doesn't matter what kind of cancer you have. Cancer sucks."

That comment led me to think he had been battered by and was resigned to his recurring cancer. I felt myself slipping into my role of twenty-six years as a vocational rehabilitation counselor. I had worked with men who had serious on-the-job injuries that left them with physical or mental limitations and the need to change careers, for many, a seemingly impossible challenge. While I helped my clients struggle to return to work, they taught me important lessons. They taught me that having a hard head is not a bad thing for many blue-collar guys. Having a hard head could save your life. May have saved this man.

I looked at the man, smiled, and said, "You must have a really strong brain and a hard head."

He smiled back, touched his shaved head, and said, "Yeah, I guess so."

I waited to see if he'd say more, but he returned to silent scrolling. As I returned to reading, I realized that I wanted to make more connections with men with cancer. The waiting room was an excellent place to do that, however brief each connection might be. And my drinking and driving helped me to an emotional space where I could listen to each man's story and demonstrate that we could talk about cancer and share our hopes and fears. I had forty more radiation treatments, forty more times to drink and drive, and do just that.

CHAPTER 25

An Elk Moment

A WEEK LATER, I FELL INTO A FUNK. IT BEGAN WHEN A bothersome bowel movement tipped me into a tantrum. When I returned from the bathroom and tried to sneak into bed without waking Mary, she asked, "Are you OK?"

"No, I'm not," I growled. "This goddam cancer has taken over my life!"

Mary rolled onto her side, put her arm around me, and whispered, "You're doing everything you can. You're taking care of your body, and I'm so proud of you. You're keeping such a positive attitude."

"Yeah, yeah, yeah," I snarled. "I do all this research so I can understand what's going on in my body, so I can feel like I have some control, so I can stay positive. But then there's questions and unknowns and nights like tonight. And there goes that positive attitude. Flushed it right down the toilet."

I sank into sulking silence and turned my head toward the window. I spotted Electric Peak, a shadowy outline against the darker sky. I searched for stars. Found one or two bright spots. Wished I could find a few bright spots in this battle with cancer.

I turned back to Mary and said, "I'm ready to go to sleep. I've got to get up early to prep for my morning radiation."

Mary slid closer and put her head on my chest. I kissed her and held her tightly. She's a bright spot.

When I walked into the Cancer Center waiting room the next morning for my next radiation shot, a gray-haired gentleman sat there. He greeted me with a hello and kind eyes. I stopped, stood near him, and returned his hello. Then, I recalled my desire to talk with more men about their cancer. Perhaps that would lift me out of the funk. Without a preamble, I asked, "What's your cancer?"

Without hesitation, he replied, "I've been fighting prostate cancer since 2003." He shook his head in disbelief.

"Oh, my, that's an incredibly long time," I sighed as I settled into the chair beside him.

He glanced at me, then looked straight ahead and dove into describing his treatment. He had his prostate removed in 2003 and was relieved to have a low PSA for years after that. Then his PSA rose, indicating the presence of cancer cells, but the doctors couldn't locate them. On hormone therapy for a couple of years, his PSA fell again. Then rose again. "The doctors tried other medications," he said, shaking his head in frustration. "But it's come back again." He touched his chest and said, "Now it's in my esophagus, and today is the first day of radiation there."

Before I could reply, a radiation therapist arrived to escort him to the treatment room. When he stood to go, I stood too, shook his hand, wished him luck, and said that I hoped we could chat again. "Me too," he said over his shoulder as he walked toward the next engagement in his unending battle.

I thought about him as I awaited my shot of radiation. Still in the early stages of my battle, I feared a story like his might become mine. I reminded myself—as Mary had—that I'm using DARE and doing everything possible to help win this battle. So are Mary and my medical team. But cancer cells are living organisms that reproduce and grow given the right conditions. There's no guarantee I'll avoid a recurrence. There's no guarantee I'll have one. Perhaps that's feeding my funk. I'm putting in all this time and energy, committing every day to using diet, attitude, rest, and exercise in a challenging fight, and I don't know how, when, or if it will end.

The following morning, the air was crisp and the sky clear as I sat on the front deck, funk still festering. Snow dusted the upper reaches of Electric Peak, reflecting the rising sun. From the direction of our back fence, a male elk bugled, loud and lovely. A moment later, another male replied from farther away. The rut, the elk mating season, was in full swing. While males collect and protect the group of females they intend to mate with, battles between males often decide who mates with whom. Perhaps the first elk said, "Hey, these are my ladies. Get lost." And the second replied, "Oh, yeah, this is my turf, so you better clear out, Bucky."

I put my journal down and stepped lightly toward the backyard and that wooden fence we had built to keep elk and other critters out. As I approached, a female elk's head appeared just above the six-foot-high fence. She stared at me with those big eyes, her nostrils flaring. I stopped and stared back.

From nearby, a male bugled, perhaps instructing her to join him and his other females. She turned her head toward the bugling and ambled in his direction.

I mounted a short stepladder that we keep beside the fence during the rut so we could sneak a peek over the fence without intruding on rut activity. The female who had stared and flared had stopped to dine on a neighbor's lawn. She was preparing her body to survive winter and possibly nurture a fetus through the harshest months of the year.

Beyond the female, I spotted a male down the gravel road that parallels our fence. He was shaking his big antlers, scanning, and bugling. During the rut, he would stay busy finding females, challenging competitors, and battling when necessary. He would rarely stop to eat. After the rut ends, he may be malnourished and weak and fall to winter or wolves. But he and the females will have fulfilled their duty and created the next generation.

I smiled, left the elk to their business, and returned to my journal. I thought about ruts. The rut these elk are in, which produces more elk, is a natural process. My rut, weeks of radiation and months of hormone therapy, is a very unnatural process. But I must attend to my rut as the elk attend to theirs. Like the male, I must fight, in my case, life-threatening cancer cells. I must endure radiation that kills the cells and hormone therapy that starves and weakens the radiation survivors. Like the female, I must nourish my body to survive this harsh time. I must give my body what it needs to make it through this cancer journey.

Once again, a life-affirming moment with nature and some of our four-legged neighbors gave me a new perspective, lifted my spirits, and freed me from the funk. I thanked the elk, closed my journal, and went into the house. It was time to get ready for the next radiation treatment.

CHAPTER 26

The Jiggle

PRONE ON THE RADIATION MACHINE'S TABLE, I AWAITED the start of my tenth treatment.

As I nestled my feet and calves into the custom-made bean bag designed during the planning session three weeks earlier, I recalled that session, which began when a nurse entered the room, handed me a mug filled with water, and said I needed to "chug the mug." Trusting that she would explain why this was essential, I chugged. When I finished, she told me to keep the mug: "You'll need it." I was unaware that this marked the beginning of an obsession with how much water I drank every day.

As I placed the empty mug in my lap, she described how that day's planning session would evolve. We would go down the hall to the treatment room, and I would lie on a table that was part of a CT machine. First, the team would take measurements to create a "bean bag-like thing" they would place under my heels and calves at the start of each upcoming radiation treatment, so that my body was always as close as possible to being in the same position. Next, I would be injected with a contrast liquid needed for that day's CT scan. Finally, the CT machine would use a series of X-rays and a computer to create detailed images, with a focus on my prostate and its neighboring rectum and bladder.

The contrast liquid was heavy and dense, and she advised me to drink plenty of water for the next two days to give my kidneys a break.

"How much is a lot?"

"Forty ounces today and sixty ounces tomorrow."

A novice at monitoring my liquid intake, I asked how my body could handle what seemed like a lot of liquid. She assured me that my kidney function was up to the task, based on the numbers from the most recent blood work.

With this return to discussing water, drinking had ascended from important to very important.

She explained that when I drank, my bladder filled and swelled. That swelling pushed much of the bladder out of the treatment field and reduced the amount of radiation hitting the bladder. The radiation therapists would monitor my bladder's fullness and position before every treatment.

"So while the bladder will move somewhat out of the way," I said, "it'll still be exposed to radiation."

She nodded and said, "The bladder is very resistant to radiation therapy. You can go to a far higher dose to the bladder than what we're going to take you to for these treatments."

She next returned to—what else?—water. When she handed me a sheet with detailed instructions for drinking and urinating before each treatment, water graduated from very important to critical.

She even told me to practice drinking correctly. I would do this by urinating and then drinking from the mug and timing to the minute how quickly my bladder filled and created the urge to purge. Practice better make perfect and put my bladder in the right shape and position for each day's radiation. If not, I would be pulled from the machine and returned to the waiting room, where I would chug more water and wait for a bladder refill and the next available slot on the radiation table.

"When you're all done this treatment," the nurse had concluded that day with a smile partially hidden by her Covid mask, "you'll be like every other man and say, 'I have never had anybody so interested in my bladder.'"

Lying on the radiation machine's table awaiting shot number ten, I was jolted from my recollection by the clicking and soft whir of the CT scan investigating—as promised—the condition and location of my bladder, prostate, and rectum. After the CT ended, I waited for the distinctive jiggling of the table—tiny movements left and right, forward and back—that I had come to expect as the therapists and the computer made the final adjustments to my body's position.

Awaiting that jiggle, I always felt nervous. Would the therapist decide that my bladder was not full enough and I needed to get off the table, drink more water, and wait for my bladder to swell? Or, because I was flirting with constipation that day and hadn't had a bowel movement, would the therapist decide that my rectum was too full and tell me that I had to empty it before radiation could begin? How could I force a bowel movement when constipated?

The table jiggled my worries away. I smiled; I'll get radiated today. What a thing to smile about.

The machine started rotating and radiating me, and I told myself to breathe, be still, relax. I held onto the little foam ring the therapists always handed me when positioning my body. Holding the blue ring on my chest kept my arms and hands out of harm's way. The machine whirred and clicked as it completed a rotation in one direction, stopped, rotated in the opposite direction, stopped, and reversed course again. After that third rotation, radiating was done.

Silence returned until a therapist entered the room and proclaimed, "All done. Let's get you off the table."

As she prepared the table for the next patient, I adjusted my scrub pants and hustled for the doorway, anxious to hit the bathroom and relieve the demanding urge from a bladder that I had been told only minutes ago had "just a light load." Whatever.

Another day of radiation was successful. That was all that mattered.

CHAPTER 27

Dreams and Cancer

As well as the daily struggles to battle cancer and handle treatment side effects, I experienced nightly struggles: troubling dreams full of conflict.

One night, in my first dream, I had taken a job in a park, perhaps Yellowstone National Park, where Mary and I had lived, worked, and volunteered. I felt lucky to have been assigned employee housing. As I walked into the bedroom, I was suddenly inside a vast aquarium, swimming along the bottom. Looking up, I saw a shark circling above me. I watched him (I somehow knew the shark was male) swim closer and closer, and then open his big mouth to show me his sharp, deadly teeth. He kept approaching until he was all I could see. As he closed in for the kill, I punched him in his long snout and yelled, "Oh, no, you don't!"

I climbed out of the aquarium, walked into the kitchen, and discovered a mountain lion. He was eating from a house cat's tiny food bowl. He lifted his head, stared at me with amber eyes, and twitched his long tail. He was big and deadly, and I knew he was preparing to attack. I ran at him, waving my arms and again yelling, "Oh, no, you don't!"

Then Mary nudged me awake. She said my grunting and struggling had awoken her. I told her about the dream. She listened and asked, "Do you want to put your head on my chest?"

I did and felt her warmth and listened to her heartbeat. Minutes later, I was asleep and dreaming again.

In the second dream, I was hiking by myself but I knew that Mary was somewhere behind me. I was picking my way along a rugged trail, over many downed trees. Then I entered a clearing and had a choice of routes. I decided to walk over to a cliff for the view. When I reached the cliff, I looked back, didn't see Mary, and thought I should retrace my steps and find her.

When I backtracked to the trail, I found it filled with wild dogs of all shapes, sizes, and colors. I stopped and stood there, wondering if I should alter my route and avoid this encounter. But Mary was somewhere back on that trail, and I would not let these wild dogs keep me from reaching her. I started toward them. They stared at me and licked their lips in hungry anticipation. I sensed danger but ran toward them, shouting, "Oh, no, you don't!"

Mary woke me again. "You were making more noise."

I told her about this dream, and she said, "There are a lot of predators after you."

The next morning, after journaling about those dreams, I decided to look for other dreams I had recorded in my journal since my prostate cancer diagnosis two months ago. I found more dreams and recurring themes: a journey, unknowns, danger, loss, and fighting. I wondered if my cancer inspired these dreams and themes. Was that possible? Had that been studied?

I headed online and first explored how dreams occur. Most, but not all, of our dreams occur during the REM (rapid eye movement) stage of sleep, according to an article by a sleep medicine physician on the Sleep Foundation website. During REM sleep, our eyes move rapidly (hence the name) behind closed eyelids, our brains are very active, our heart rate increases, and our breathing becomes irregular. We experience a loss of muscle tone, and that's helpful: we can't move around in our beds as much as we do in our dreams.

The National Library of Medicine presents a study of the sleep and dreams reported by cancer patients in focus groups. Some participants were scheduled to begin or were undergoing treatment for cancers, including prostate cancer. Others were in post-treatment follow-up. The participants had experienced a variety of treatments, including surgery, chemotherapy, radiation therapy, hormonal therapy, molecularly targeted therapy, and multimodal treatments. The researchers transcribed and analyzed the focus group discussions to identify significant themes.

Their analysis found that participants reported causes of sleep disturbance common in other populations. However, participants also reported causes that could be unique to cancer populations, including abnormal dreams, night sweats, and problems with sleep positioning. Worry or fear related to diagnosis, prognosis, or recurrence was another major cancer-related theme.

I found little scientific evidence to support the idea that a dream's content is related to a specific health issue, such as cancer. However, I found experts who stated that dreams can help us access things we're not consciously aware of. For example, the director of the Dream & Nightmare Laboratory at the University of Montreal in Quebec told *Discover Magazine* that dreams and nightmares are "dipsticks" into our unconscious and can tell us something needs attention.

The dreams I was attending to revealed that I felt attacked, as Mary had noted, by predators. Having predators as the main characters made sense. I had spent time observing predators in Yellowstone as they took the prey they needed to survive. Their actions were natural and necessary, not negative. In Yellowstone, everyone eats.

But in my dreams, I was the prey. I figured that prostate cancer was portrayed by the predators I faced and feared. I was fighting back, but didn't know if I would win. If I didn't win, I could lose my life and connection to the people and places I love. That life-threatening dream content seemed consistent with days of facing a life-threatening disease.

Whatever their source, my intense dreams revealed that this fight was more ferocious than I allowed myself to admit during the day. At night, during REM sleep, my dreams took charge and painted inescapable pictures of high stakes and deep danger. Those dreams scared me, but also reminded me and motivated me to keep up the fight in the days and months ahead.

CHAPTER 28

Lines of Defense

AFTER TWO WEEKS OF RADIATION AND TWO MONTHS OF hormone therapy, the first line of defense in this battle, Mary and I were making headway on building our second line of defense: the DARE approach.

In the months since radically reshaping our diet, Mary and I had each lost eighteen pounds.

Mary recorded and limited her daily calorie intake; she didn't want to regain weight. I, on the other fork-filled hand, wanted to regain. I ate without limits — as long as I consumed cancer-fighting foods.

We stopped eating meat after reading more research. With determination overcoming sadness, we gave away a small freezer full of our share of an elk a neighbor had taken locally. The contents of our refrigerator had also changed. Processed foods were out. Unprocessed and fresh were in. We stocked more seafood for its cancer-fighting qualities.

While eating well, I worked on my attitude. Unlike diet, where I measured a meal's nutritional and cancer-fighting value, attitude was much more challenging to quantify but equally important.

Feeling relieved and comfortable with how treatment was progressing helped me maintain a life-affirming attitude. I felt positive and hopeful. I felt confident in my medical team's skills. I felt cared for; the staff was conscientious, friendly, and willing to answer my many questions.

However, the team could not definitively answer some of the scariest ones: How will the treatment go? How strongly will side effects impact daily life? What will my PSA score show about the presence of cancer cells after radiation? What is the likelihood of a recurrence? Those questions could only be answered over time; trying to force an answer would be a waste of time.

But I believed that when questions and concerns arose, I had to face them, not keep them locked inside, so they kept me awake at night or filled my dreams with dangerous predators. I aimed to expose my feelings to the light of day by sharing them with Mary, my family, and friends, sometimes finding tears, sometimes joy.

I also continued visiting my paper therapist to help maintain a positive attitude and reduce stress. Some days, I didn't feel like journaling, but I pushed myself to put pen to paper, to let words appear and take me where they may.

Unlike attitude, rest was easy to measure. My fitness watch and its phone app told me how long and well I slept each night. I started using the watch when hormone therapy began. I found my nighttime sleep to be consistent in length and restorative quality. My after-lunch naps varied in length because I didn't set an alarm; I let my body decide when to wake up.

Though I was getting ample rest, my fatigue had increased. For example, I slept a little longer than usual one night. After breakfast, I completed some less-than-strenuous tasks to prepare the yard for the fast-approaching winter. By lunch, I was yawning, sighing, sagging, and eager to stop. While fixing lunch, I felt so tired that standing at the kitchen counter challenged me. Finally, I collapsed in a chair and ate.

After lunch, I said "Good night" to Mary as she strummed her ukulele in her music studio. I went into our bedroom, undressed, and giggled as I slid between a fleece blanket and a down comforter. I read for ten minutes before dropping my phone and glasses onto the comforter and succumbing. About twenty minutes later, I awoke but stayed in bed, delighting in the softness of the covers and the day's silence. Before treatment began, such a delay in putting my feet back on the floor was unusual.

Finally, I ordered myself to get up and get busy. I went to the front yard and finished another thirty minutes of easy yard work. Then I went into the house to make a cup of sugar-free espresso. As I worked the espresso machine, I felt as tired as I had before lunch, yet I had been up for less than an hour. And that, as I understood it, was one definition of fatigue: feeling tired even after ample rest. While this was an expected treatment side effect, I wondered and worried how much the fatigue would increase in the remaining weeks of radiation and months of hormone therapy.

Although fighting fatigue, I had increased my exercise regimen after reading extensive research on the importance of exercise in combating cancer. In addition to hiking, walking, running, and exercise biking, I included mowing the lawn as a workout. The data from my fitness watch showed that by rejecting the self-propelled mode and pushing the mower with speed and consistency, my heart rate increased to that of an aerobic walk. I would take a workout in any form, especially if I could be outside.

But fatigue challenged exercise. One day, after a morning radiation treatment, I planned to run on the inviting foot trails adjacent to the Cancer Center. I had even worn my running shoes and those new sweatpants I had modeled for Mary. But as I left the building and walked through the parking lot, I muttered aloud, "I don't feel like running. Don't have the energy." A few steps later, "Oh, come on, Rick. It's a beautiful day, the trails are lovely, and you need another workout to make your weekly numbers."

Spurred by that need, I stepped onto a gravel trail, began to jog, and encouraged myself by speaking in a soft coaching voice: "Come on, you can do this. Your body needs it. It'll feel good when you're done."

My body countered with an immediate non-verbal reply: *I'm tired and sluggish! I don't want to jog! Stop this right now!* My body stressed its demand by making my heart pound and my lungs gasp. But I pushed on because I had learned over the years that during the first twenty minutes of most workouts, my body would do all it could to make me stop. I had come to call this the "terrible twenty."

After struggling through that terrible twenty, my endocannabinoid system and endorphins kicked in, my mood improved, and I felt capable of tackling some hills. On one particularly long and steep hill, I had to stop running and start walking. Though I blamed my laggard pace on treatment fatigue, my inner high achiever still scolded me for coming up short.

But after I arrived home and checked the data from my fitness watch, I was surprised and pleased to find that I had run at a speed close to a pre-treatment pace. As I stared at the data, I realized that my challenge would not only be overcoming actual treatment-induced fatigue, I would also need to dispel the false belief that I was too tired to exercise.

When I busted that mental barrier that day, my body showed it could still perform. I felt confident that diet, attitude, and rest had helped me. It remained to be seen how my body's abilities would decrease as the months of treatment continued. But I intended to stay proactive and use DARE to build my second line of defense.

CHAPTER 29

Lesson from Sacagawea

WHEN WE ARRIVED AT THE SACAJAWEA PEAK TRAILHEAD, after an eighty-mile drive, the parking lot was full. As we shouldered into our daypacks, Mary scanned the cars and people and asked, "You still want to do this?"

"I do," I said, excited to be in nature again, even though we preferred to hike where we saw few people.

Without further discussion, we followed the broad and well-worn trail into the shade of a conifer forest. Soon, the forest thinned, and we took in the pointed peaks around us. A short while later, we were above the tree line. We stopped and, hand in hand, turned a full circle on a ridge between two peaks.

"Wow," Mary said, "I'm so glad we're doing this."

"Me too." The beauty surrounding me overcame the weeks of tension inside me. I settled into nature and outside myself.

I was ten weeks into treatment, and some of the side effects, especially fatigue and hot flashes, were troubling and obvious. But one significant side effect was surprisingly subtle. Since subjecting my body to hormone therapy and radiation, I limited what I did outside the house: I had become a captive of the bathroom. That, in turn, reduced my needed time in nature.

That trade-off became clear to me after Mary and I spoke with a friend who had just hiked up Sacajawea Peak. Listening to his description and recommendation made me eager to do the same. Then, my agitated bladder and bowels chimed in: it was time to go. As I hustled down the hallway, I wondered how often and where I would relieve myself above tree line on that peak's exposed slopes.

This challenge to my gastrointestinal system, what I called "the GIs," was to be expected. The National Cancer Institute stated on its website that combining hormone therapy with radiation can increase some of radiation's side effects. My shots of radiation generated numerous side effects, including the GIs. My concurrent hormone therapy increased them.

Worse yet: "Many of the side effects of ongoing hormone therapy also become stronger the longer a man takes hormone therapy." My eighteen months of hormone therapy, a standard approach for my aggressive cancer, qualified as a long time and would produce its own batch of increasingly strong side effects. Troubled times ahead.

A few days after our friend's recommendation, I talked with Mary early in the morning about Sacajawea Peak and my GIs. "I've been thinking about the hike and being outside. But I've realized how attached I've become to staying near a bathroom." Mary looked puzzled. "Think about it: for the most part, I'm only out of the house for an hour or so when I take a walk or run. So, I'm not sure I want to try a four-hour hike."

"It's OK," Mary said with concern but no irritation. "I understand. Whatever works for you works for me."

I felt relieved and thankful. Her support helped me decide. I took her hand and said, "But I'm willing to try. Let's go."

She smiled, and we collected the gear that was now on our backs as we entered a series of switchbacks that climbed a steep, rocky slope. Sometimes, the rocks were dangerously loose, and I had to focus on balance and foot placement. Other times, the footing was satisfactory, and I could gaze with amazement at the subtle streaks of white, beige, black, and brown decorating the slope.

Looking ahead, I watched Mary climb and marveled at how small she appeared in this giant landscape. I was rocked from my rubbernecking by the beeping of my phone—an off-route alert from the hiking app. I stopped, opened the phone, and oriented the phone's map to the peaks around us. I slapped my forehead and chuckled when I realized we should have turned in the opposite direction at the last trail junction. Now, instead of heading toward 9,654-foot Sacajawea Peak, named in honor of a Shoshone woman who, at seventeen years of age, had worked as a guide and interpreter for the Lewis and Clark expedition, we were climbing toward the summit of 9,550-foot Pomp Peak, named in honor of her son.

When I caught up with Mary and explained our wrong turn, she looked around, pointed at Sacajawea Peak, and said, "I don't want to scramble back down this rocky slope we just struggled up to, then go up that rocky slope."

"Me neither. Let's keep climbing. Who cares where we're going or where we stop? The mom or the son is fine with me. We're out here, and that's all that matters."

As we continued, I sometimes had to grab onto large boulders to help keep my footing and balance. We soon came to a spot with a bit of flat space and enchanting views of mountains, both nearby and distant. After we stopped to catch our breath, we decided this would be our lunch spot.

Fixated on the view as I nibbled on a banana, I felt a wave of nausea and said softly to Mary, "I don't think I should stay here very long."

"What's happening?"

"I just feel a little nauseated and don't know what that means."

"Okay," Mary said, wolfing down the last of an energy bar. "I'm just finishing up."

"Thanks for understanding."

"No prob! I'm just glad we're out here. This is exactly what I wanted to do today."

"Me too. I'm so glad I didn't let my nervousness stop me. It would have been so easy to bail out of doing this."

"Yeah," Mary said. "There's a lesson in that."

We decided to pack up and descend; we wouldn't reach either peak today, which was fine with us both.

We used our hiking poles to help maintain our footing and balance. Walking became more manageable once we left the rugged trail and reentered the forest; I had time to reflect on today's lesson.

As side effects had increased, I had slowly and subtly limited my time in nature by staying close to home, near a bathroom, and in a comfortable routine. On that hike, I overcame my resistance and broke out of my routine. Everything went well.

I looked forward to breaking away again; being in nature was a personal prescription in my Lifestyle Medicine.

CHAPTER 30

Worst or Challenging?

TWO WEEKS AFTER THAT HEALING HIKE, THE WORST OF times snuck up on me. I was halfway through radiation and deep into hormone therapy. In the morning, during a strength-and-stretch workout, I struggled to complete my usual reps, even with reduced weights. I felt weaker and less energetic than I had the last time I did the same workout. My mind wanted to keep my body strong and healthy. My body wanted to snuggle on the sofa and read. But I persisted, panting and sweating in a battle of mind over muscle.

Later in the day, I grimaced at a sharp burning pain in my stomach. It didn't feel like muscle pain. It felt like gastrointestinal trouble. Oh, no, more GIs! The pain erupted off and on over the next few hours and reached an apex that felt as if someone had punched me in the stomach. When the pain subsided, I worried it would return. It did.

By the end of the day, all I wanted to do was crawl into bed and sleep away the pain. But during the first four hours of the night, I was jolted awake six times by painful movement and growling in my bowels. What a night!

I awoke to a gray, cloud-covered morning that matched my dark wondering about what ailed my digestive system. My GIs were much worse than they had been when Mary and I had hiked partway up Pomp Peak. I assumed that I was experiencing the increased side effects produced by the one-two punch of radiation and hormone therapy.

For the next fifteen days, I struggled with and journaled about those GIs and the worst of times. I wrote about urinating way too often and bouncing between diarrhea and constipation. Mary and I thought the problem might be our high-fiber diet; we shifted to low-fiber. The GIs got worse. We returned to high-fiber. As some troubles left and others arrived, I had ample opportunity to wonder and worry. What's happening to my body? Why's it happening? What can I do?

One thing I could do was talk to my team members: the radiation therapists, the nurses, and the oncologist. Each listened, nodded, and empathized. I learned, once again, that everybody's body responds differently to radiation. Perhaps these GIs were my body's response.

I felt a little optimistic when the oncologist told me that I had reached the point in my radiation where "the boost" would begin. During the boost, the team would zoom in on the prostate, shrink the irradiated area, and reduce exposure to my bladder and rectum. They said the boost *could eventually* decrease my GIs.

Meanwhile, I also had to deal with emotional side effects. One morning, Mary and I were showering together when she asked how my night had gone. When I started to explain my worst of times, my voice broke, and tears took over. Mary's eyes told me she saw me crying, even with the shower water running down my face. I pulled her to me, wrapped my arms around her, and leaned my wet head against hers.

She whispered her mantra in my ear, "It's okay, you're going to get through this." I nodded, sniffled, and held her tighter as she added, "It's good to cry. Just let it out."

I didn't try to speak or stop crying for what felt like a long time. Finally, I released her and turned my face into the shower stream, letting the water wash away the tears, the sadness, the fear, and the uncertainty that plagued me during those worst of times.

Eventually, as the days and the boost continued, the worst of times faded. I'm not sure I did anything to help them go away. Instead, as my team had speculated, my bladder and rectum had been struggling with the effects of radiation, and as the boost reduced their exposure, the troubles decreased.

One morning, I journaled about experiencing no GIs during the night and the joy of feeling almost normal. The day was also distress-free. So was a second when I felt brave enough to go for a gentle jog on a favorite trail a few miles from home. I was away from the house for a couple of hours! A third day went off without a hitch or a sprint down the hall. As the GIs slipped into the past, I wondered if the worst of times was over.

Thinking back on that time, I realize I made a poor word choice. Calling it "the worst of times" evoked a sense of resignation and acceptance that things were bad. There was little call to action other than waiting for things to improve.

Calling it "the most challenging of times" would have been better. A challenge is something to accept or avoid—I have a choice. I chose to take that challenge, do my best under the circumstances, and work for improvement during the most challenging of times.

CHAPTER 31

Cancer-Caused Changes

ONE AFTERNOON, THREE MONTHS INTO TREATMENT, I
opened my mind and heart to cancer-caused changes.
Mary and I were at the kitchen peninsula sorting the
day's mail. She handed me an envelope, and I was surprised and pleased to see the return address of an Oregon
friend. I pulled out a greeting card. The photo on the
card's front of some bison — my favorite Yellowstone
neighbors — walking across the rainbow-colored edge of
one of my favorite Yellowstone thermal features brought
a huge smile.

Opening the card, I was touched by the inscription:
"The men's retreat that you got started years ago lives
on. We, the men of this weekend's retreat, Thank You!"

As I scanned the card, I was even happier to find
inscriptions and signatures from men I recalled from
those retreats when we lived in Oregon. Noticing that
all the writing was in the same black ink, I imagined
the card and pen being passed around the circle of men

I had been a part of for many years. A circle where I learned a great deal about what it means to be a man. A circle I miss.

As I read how the men wished me well and sometimes still felt my presence at a retreat, tears flowed. When I put the card down to wipe my eyes, Mary slid over and held me. When I could finally speak, I whispered through sniffles, "Another circle closing." All those years later, those caring men had reached out to share their feelings, thoughts, and thanks at a time when I was deep into fighting cancer and desperate for such support.

Standing in the kitchen of our Montana home, thinking about those Oregon friends at a retreat, I felt lonely and lacking in male connections. I longed for deeper, more intimate male relationships like I had enjoyed with some of those men. Achieving that would not be easy. I would have to understand what was important to me, what was not, and who I was now as a man. I would have to take risks, share my feelings with certain men, and see who reciprocated.

Card in hand, an image came to mind. I had just opened a box filled with puzzle pieces. The box cover showed no picture of how the finished puzzle was supposed to look. Instead, a caption read, "You'll know when the puzzle looks right." I dumped the pieces onto a tabletop. There were so many to move around and try to fit together. Some didn't fit. Some did. But with time and persistence and courage inspired by cancer, I would strive to put the pieces together, create a clear image of the man I had become, and share it with other men before this final quarter of my life ended.

A few days later, as I walked around our backyard, I walked right into another cancer-caused change: an intense focus on the frailty and finality of life.

A sliver of the moon hung low in the west, sometimes obscured by passing clouds. The sun was near the horizon. Gusts of wind chilled me. The forecast called for snow and high winds—late fall in Montana.

I looked at the conifers we had planted. Our green friends were entering their most challenging time, especially that one young pine Mary had said weeks ago was dying, a condition I still refused to accept. I walked over and stood in front of the ailing pine. I brushed a branch now full of red and brown needles; many spilled to the needle-covered ground.

I had tried my best to save that tree, watering and paying more attention to it than its neighbors. To no avail, the green kept turning red. Finally, and painfully, the truth was obvious: this green friend was gone.

I walked to the workshop and grabbed a saw. I returned to the tree and stood there, rubbing my thumb along the points of the saw's teeth, flinching at their sharpness. I whispered an apology to the tree for failing to save it. I thanked the tree for the short time we had together. I grabbed a red-orange branch at waist level and shook it like I would a friend's hand. More needles fell. I dropped to my knees, leaned in, and took the saw to the thin trunk. I winced as I started the cut, but continued until the tree fell, creating a tiny red and brown cloud. I cut the tree into shorter pieces and placed each in a big black bucket that I drove to the local recycling center. I hefted the bucket from the back of the car, carried it to a massive pile of fellow fallen trees, and gently dumped it with a sad goodbye.

I felt awkward carrying on about that tree. It was one of many and could be replaced. But my feelings were real. Part of my sadness stemmed from the love of landscaping that Mary and I share. We have planted and nurtured trees and shrubs for many years, and the payoff has always been watching them mature and flourish.

But another part of my sadness was cancer-caused. That pine showed the first troubling signs of dying just after I was diagnosed with aggressive prostate cancer. It started to morph from green to red as I researched the dangers of my life-threatening disease. It became a red symbol of death as I began hormone therapy and radiation, and worried about what was in store for me. Finally, my failure to save the pine became a painful preview of the possibility of treatment failing to save me.

Cancer had brought my mortality center stage and made me sensitive to death, my own, and that of the pine.

CHAPTER 32

Ring the Bell

"TODAY'S YOUR LAST DAY," THE RADIATION THERAPIST SAID as she approached me in the waiting room. Her eyes hinted at a smile hidden by her COVID-required mask.

"It sure is!" I exclaimed, standing and slapping my thigh.

"Are you going to ring the bell?" she asked as we walked past it on our way to the treatment area and the last of my radiation treatments.

"You bet I am!"

This bell-ringing tradition began at the MD Anderson Cancer Center in Texas in 1996, when Irve Le Moyne, a rear admiral in the U.S. Navy, told his doctor he wanted to follow a Navy tradition of ringing a bell to signify a job done. Le Moyne brought a brass bell to his last cancer treatment, rang it, and donated it to the Center. The Center mounted the bell with a wall plaque explaining its use. Patients took to ringing it when their treatment ended. The practice spread to other cancer centers.

A paper published in the *Canadian Oncology Nursing Journal* found that this ritual creates a sense of community among cancer patients, helps them mark a significant milestone, and provides a sense of self-determination as they finish treatment.

I felt all three as I looked at the therapist and, with a smile behind my mask, asked, "Do I have to have a full bladder and empty rectum to ring the bell?"

She laughed. "No, you can have both as empty as you like."

"I can't believe how many conversations I've had in the last nine weeks about my bladder and rectum," I said as we stopped at the computer station just outside the treatment room.

She laughed again and studied the computer screen. Well-trained after forty-three previous stops here, I recited my birth date. For the last time, she confirmed that I was the patient on the screen and accompanied me into the treatment room. I hopped onto the treatment table, and she and a male therapist adjusted my position. As they worked, the second staffer said, "Last time."

"And I'm so happy it is!"

"Are you going to ring the bell?"

"I wouldn't miss it!" I said, clapping my hands.

They finished adjusting my position and left the room. The machine whirred and clicked and began its first rotation, checking to see that I had a full bladder and an empty rectum. As always, I told my nervous self to relax. A moment later, there was the jiggle. I'm in!

The final rotations and final radiation treatment began and ended.

The male staffer reentered the room and shouted, "Party time!"

"Yahoo! Will you two join me?" I shouted as I sat up.

"Sure will. We'll give you time to change into your regular clothes, and we'll meet you at the bell," he said.

And so they did, along with most of the nurses and front desk staff. I felt cared for and grateful. I thanked them for helping me through these nine challenging weeks of radiation. As they smiled and looked on, I rang the bell. Job done.

At home later in the day, I realized that with radiation finished, another milestone, another decision awaited: Should I continue hormone therapy? I needed to decide soon; my second injection was just a week away.

As always, I wanted the best information to make the best decision. I went online to research hormone therapy again. I even studied its history. In the 1940s, a researcher found that cancer that had spread beyond the prostate responded to treatment that reduced androgens, a group of sex hormones that includes testosterone. During the 1960s to the 1980s, researchers developed specific drugs to block or reduce testosterone. One of those was Lupron, the drug used in my hormone therapy. Lupron was first approved by the FDA in 1985 and is heavily used in the United States.

A 2001 scientific paper published on the National Library of Medicine website reported that three scientific trials have shown that combining hormone therapy with radiation improved the survival rate of men with pros-tate cancer. This one-two-punch has been the standard of care for a quarter of a century, especially for men like me with aggressive prostate cancer.

Given that supportive history and the appropriate-ness of hormone therapy, what was my problem with just saying yes to the drug?

Pondering that question, I scrolled through lists of the treatment's substantial side effects. Unfortunately, I was not sure how many of those side effects I had expe-rienced in the months since hormone therapy began. The intense side effects from radiation had taken all my time and attention from the possible side effects of hormone therapy. Except, of course, for erectile dysfunction and loss of interest in sex. Those two appeared as soon as my testosterone level fell after the first injection of Lupron and weeks before radiation began. As those two side effects eradicated our sex life, Mary and I mourned the loss.

If any side effects would lead me to just say no to the drug, erectile dysfunction and loss of interest in sex would top the list. Right behind them would be the loss of muscle mass and bone density that could occur as the months of hormone therapy went on and on and on.

But as I sat at the computer, a different thought crossed my mind: I want to do everything possible to fight this cancer. I never want to face defeat and sadly say, "If only I had done…" Instead, if I eventually fall to cancer, I want to be able to stand proud and proclaim, "I did everything I could to beat this. I have no regrets."

Viewed from that perspective, I made another life-affirming decision: I would complete hormone therapy; it has worked for many years for many men. I would take the injections.

CHAPTER 33

A Passing

I RECEIVED NEWS THAT DICK, A FRIEND OF MINE IN OREGON, had passed away. He lived to be eighty-nine. Some years ago, while driving his car, he had a head-on collision with a cement truck that left him — an active athlete — in a wheelchair. But limited physical ability didn't stop him from mentally and socially engaging with life. He took classes in writing, and that's where I met him.

Over the years, we helped each other write and publish books. As we grew closer, I would come to the long-term care home where he lived, and, rain or snow, but usually Oregon rain, roll him in his wheelchair to a nearby coffee shop. Over coffee and a sweet treat (I was still a sugar addict then), we would talk and laugh about a myriad of topics as other customers, particularly kids, walked by and snuck a peek at Dick with his big smile, hearty laugh, and flowing white hair.

After Mary and I moved to Montana, I visited Dick when we returned to Oregon to see friends and family.

Each time, Dick and I picked up where we left off, a true measure of our friendship. Then COVID hit; I made fewer trips, and Dick's facility was often locked down. We connected less and less.

When I learned he was gone, I felt sad and guilty because we had lost touch. I wished I had made the effort to tell him again that he was a friend, a mentor, and an inspiration.

My reaction to Dick's passing prompted me to reconnect with three other Oregon friends I had lost touch with. In an email, I wrote to each about Dick's passing. I described how I had faced my mortality in the months since my prostate cancer diagnosis and, while doing so, had realized the importance of staying in touch. I told each friend how I had enjoyed our moments together and how each had inspired me at different times. I ended by writing that I would love a reply, but one way or the other, I wanted to thank each for the friendship and the years we had enjoyed.

Dick's passing also pushed me to finally tell the readers of *Love the Wild* and *Save the Wild*, my earlier Substack publications, about another passing: the demise of my writing about and advocating for wolves, bison, and wild lands.

In both publications, I explained how I had been diagnosed and was four months into treatment and coping with side effects. I wrote that in addition to the physical leg of this journey, there was a life-changing emotional leg: I no longer had the heart to post. I hadn't stopped writing; I wrote every day. But my focus had changed. Writing had become journaling about facts and feelings, a visit to my paper therapist. While that approach was essential, it was not about loving the wild or saving the wild. It was about loving family and friends and saving my life.

I still loved being in the wild — might even enjoy each trip, each dose of nature's medicine, more since diagnosis. I still respected wolves and treasured my days of observing and photographing them. I was still concerned about saving them, but numerous conservation organizations had committed to fighting the battle during my decade as an advocate. I saw myself as no longer needed.

I thanked readers of both publications for their years of commenting and sharing thoughts and feelings. For supporting and encouraging me to keep writing and advocating even when it seemed we lost every battle. Without their support, being shouted down at local meetings by angry neighbors who wanted to kill, not protect, wolves, being frustrated during visits with unresponsive Montana legislators and Fish and Game staff, and being ignored by senators and representatives in Washington, D.C., would have driven me to the sidelines.

I ended by announcing that I would no longer post to either publication. Perhaps I would return someday to Substack with postings about this journey into the wilds of cancer. I didn't know what the future would bring.

Many readers shared heartfelt replies. Some brought me to tears. I was surprised to learn how many had either battled cancer or helped a friend or loved one do so. Some were in the battle even as they wrote. An over-riding message was to take care of myself and return when and if I could. I felt so supported by many people I had never met in person.

With that post, I interacted with readers in a different way than I did pre-diagnosis. For the previous ten years, I had presented myself as an advocate for wildlife and wild lands. I had advocated strongly, for example, to help create situations and places where wolves were welcome or at least accepted. Where we could coexist with wolves—live and let live.

But post-diagnosis, I saw myself becoming a *feeling* advocate, working to identify and nurture relationships where feelings were welcome or at least accepted. Where we could comfortably coexist with our feelings—share and let share. I wanted to find others—especially men—to go deeper with.

I was glad that Dick's passing led me to contact three old friends and seek deeper connections. I was encouraged when I heard back from one of those friends immediately. He wrote, "I'm responding with damp, misty eyes to your beautiful message...Your words fit so well with a stream of recent experiences, which remind me of the profound joy and pain that make us human."

I looked forward to going deeper with him. And maybe even others.

CHAPTER 34

Meet Your Bear

Last night I had another memorable dream. Mary and I were hiking nervously on a Yellowstone trail bounded on both sides by thick, leafy vegetation that dwarfed us. We knew this was a perfect place to encounter a grizzly bear. I happened to be in front, and when I came around a slight bend, I spotted the grizzly we feared meeting. The griz had not sensed our presence and was standing calmly on all fours in the trail just ahead, looking away from us. I stopped and whispered to Mary, "Bear." As practiced, we began backing up slowly and quietly. We didn't want to surprise the bear into feeling the need to defend itself.

As we retreated, the bear sensed our presence and ran away to the right of the trail. When it disappeared from view, I felt relieved and thought we might be out of danger. We stopped, and I turned to face Mary, fear as evident on her face as I'm sure it was on mine.

Then, behind her, I heard running paws pounding and dried leaves rustling. Scared, I hoped it wasn't the bear. That hope died quickly as the griz charged around a curve, heading straight for me. It knocked me to the ground and onto my back. The bear then lay on top of me, its massive chest pressing on my chest and stomach. Its big snout, nostrils flaring after the running, pressed against my chin. I felt the moistness of the nose and smelled the bear's wild, hot breath.

To my surprise, the griz didn't bite or claw me. Instead, it watched me with its big eyes wide open and intense. I averted my eyes, not wanting to lock into a challenging stare. The bear lifted a massive claw, reached toward my face, and pushed gently on my forehead with the point of one claw. I felt like a friend had tapped me on my shoulder and tried to encourage me with, "Oh, come on, Rick, get it together."

But I was still terrified. I looked off to the left and focused on an object that had appeared magically in the air: a round, copper-colored shield the size of the bear's big head. Around the outer circumference of the shield were raised words. Though I don't recall any of the words, I remember that focusing on them, reading them, and absorbing them was a calming meditation. That focus on the words, I somehow knew, would protect me from the bear, would keep me safe until the griz realized I was no danger and left me unharmed on the trail.

I awoke from the dream, sweating, my heart banging. I lay on my back, emitted a long moan, and stared at the ceiling. When Mary rustled beside me, I whispered, "Are you awake?"

"Yes."

"I had another nightmare."

"I know," she said. "I felt you moving around and muttering. You want to talk about it?" As I described the dream, Mary listened in silence. Then she said, "You were meeting your bear again."

"Huh," I said, surprised. "That's true."

"Meet your bear" was a phrase that originated years ago after we encountered a backpacker along a trail in Yellowstone's Lamar Valley. When we stopped to chat, he told us he was excited to be hiking eleven miles back to a campsite where he had seen a grizzly four times while camping there a week earlier. He said the griz had seemed to know he was there but had not bothered him. I asked if he thought he might see the griz again. "I sure hope so," he said with a grin.

After the hiker resumed his trek to the grizzly, Mary and I talked about him. He looked and sounded like a competent and experienced backpacker, but he was returning to a potentially dangerous situation that had scared him just days earlier. We decided he was going to meet his bear. That phrase, "meet your bear," became our shorthand for intentionally going to places—mental, physical, or emotional—that scared us.

Lying in bed, we began decoding the dream and the bear encounter. While fighting prostate cancer, we were in a scary place, a perfect place to meet my bear. Perhaps the bear represented big, bad cancer coming to attack me and take me away. But, no, my heart and mind had sent me a benevolent bear, one that didn't want to harm me. Instead, the griz's gentle tap on my forehead encouraged me to get myself together. Right after that tap, I looked off and saw the shield and words. The words calmed and strengthened me, even as I lay there with a bear on my chest. The words, we figured, represented my journaling, the visits to my paper therapist, about this journey into the wilds of prostate cancer.

As I looked ahead to a long grind of twelve more months of hormone therapy, my heart and mind had delivered a dream bear to remind me that journaling would help me travel this scary path, where I couldn't see the dangers that lurked ahead. Journaling would be my shield and help me survive this encounter with cancer, this meeting with my bear.

CHAPTER 35

Routinizing

REACHING THE SIX-MONTH MILESTONE OF CONVENTIONAL medical treatment felt like a landmark, so I decided to review the journal entries I had written during that period. When I did, one conclusion stood out: Since treatment began, I had routinized my diet, rest, and exercise—three key components of our DARE approach.

Mary guided us in establishing a dietary routine. She's a researcher, cook, and baker extraordinaire. She spent many hours researching the cancer-fighting properties of specific foods, collecting recipes with cancer-fighting properties, and modifying other recipes to incorporate more cancer-fighting ingredients. We became primarily vegetarian, with some vegan meals and seafood. Because of Mary's efforts, my body received the necessary nutrition at every meal and snack to fight my cancer and support exercise and rest.

I routinized rest by slipping under the covers each night around 9 p.m. and sliding out around 5 a.m. I called this my new nine-to-five shift. Just like at work, those eight hours of sleep were interrupted. I got up two to three times to urinate each night.

Months ago, before my radiation treatment ended, my oncologist described how my "not-too-bright" bladder buddy would respond to radiation with more nighttime urination. He said those nighttime visits would decrease once radiation ended. My urologist, on the other hand, predicted increased urination would be a long-term radiation side effect. Was I experiencing a preview of that? Or was my night time busyness simply a function of being in my 70s?

I found an article on a trusted source, the Cleveland Clinic website. The article quotes a Clinic urologist as saying, "In fact, it's normal for a 60-year-old man to get up once, a 70-year-old man to get up twice, and an 80-year-old man to get up three times a night." That estimation, though perhaps too simplified, fit with me and the men I had talked to about nightly walks down the hall.

I decided to keep a record of my nightly busyness. Once hormone therapy ended, I would discuss my data and concerns with the oncologist and urologist and hear what each had to say. Then, the medical team, Mary, and I could decide what, if anything, we needed to do next.

As I researched sleep and recorded my sleep patterns, I gained a deeper understanding of sleep's importance, particularly in two of its stages: light sleep and deep sleep. Light sleep occurs when heartbeat, breathing, and body temperature decrease while the muscles and brain relax.

Deep sleep goes beyond relaxing; it restores. During deep sleep, the body physically recovers from the day, the immune system recharges, and the mind and heart process the day's learning and emotions.

"There are no guidelines for the amount of deep sleep a person needs, though most adults spend about 10% to 20% of each night in the deep sleep," the Sleep Foundation stated on its website. My fitness watch tracked my deep sleep and reported I was usually within that range.

I was encouraged to exercise five to six days a week by my love of being active in nature, as well as Mary's. Living in Gardiner helped, too. We had so many places to explore and enjoy that working out meant having fun together for hours as we followed animal trails or huffed and puffed to a summit, stopping often to catch our breath and gawk at the view.

My fitness watch app provided abundant data on each workout, from heartbeats per minute to the impact of the effort on my body and fitness level. I recorded the data so I could compare my body's response to each workout and over time. The app also rated my exercise as "good workout," "high," or "overreaching." I hit overreaching most of the time—not surprising for an overachiever who lives where hiking and cross-country skiing are accessible, enjoyable, physically demanding, and time-consuming.

At first, I worried about overreaching and pushing my body too hard. But I decided that regardless of what the app said, my body had the final word—if I listened. So I paid attention and looked for messages my body might send: dull aches, sharp pains, stiff joints. Even with all that overreaching with my now 74-year-old body, no aches, pains, or stiffness had sidelined me. I figured that including two weekly strength-and-stretch workouts, as well as stretching after vigorous aerobic workouts, must help. In the past, I was never much for stretching and often sidelined as a result.

Routinizing diet, rest, and exercise was one thing. Staying committed to following those routines was another, and that was where attitude came in. Over the last six months, my biggest revelation about attitude was that our DARE approach was not just for use during treatment. Since my oncologist had estimated a fifty percent chance of recurrence, once treatment finally ended, my diet, exercise, and rest routines would graduate from being my second line of defense to being my first.

I would continue the DARE approach to keep any surviving cancer cells at a disadvantage. While that statement is easy to write, it could be a challenge to implement every day—especially if I felt as if I had won this battle because follow-up showed low PSA numbers that revealed no significant cancer cell activity. How much harm, I might wonder, could there be in adding a couple of sugars to my coffee? Did I still need to maintain eight hours of restorative sleep every night? Why force myself to exercise when I didn't feel like it?

Maintaining the attitude that encouraged me to use those routines for the rest of my life would help me make my body a hostile environment for prostate cancer cells and a haven for healthy cells. That was no small goal, but six months into treatment, I felt prepared and ready to DARE to achieve it.

CHAPTER 36

Low Testosterone

Last night, while watching a tv drama, mary and i broke down in tears at a touching scene of a funeral with a military honor guard for a homeless Korean War veteran. He had died from exposure during a long, cold winter night spent sleeping on a park bench near the Vietnam Memorial in Washington, D.C. While it was not unusual for Mary to cry during sad scenes, it was rare for me. Even though that was not the first time I had shed tears since my diagnosis of aggressive prostate cancer, I felt awkward and embarrassed.

A few moments after the scene ended, I asked Mary, "I wonder if I'm so emotional because of my lack of testosterone?" We chuckled at that question as we wiped our eyes and recovered.

More than six months into hormone therapy, my testosterone level was extremely low—close to zero. No surprise; that was the therapy's objective. Since prostate cancer cells feed on testosterone, eliminating that food source would starve and weaken them. That's the good news. The bad news is that testosterone is essential. If I weren't in hormone therapy and my testosterone level had fallen to such a low level, I would be a candidate for several medical treatments to raise the level.

The next day, I decided to research the effects of low testosterone caused by hormone therapy. I found many reputable websites that repeated numerous side effects I was aware of, including hot flashes, fatigue, anxiety, depression, irritability, insomnia, erectile dysfunction, loss of interest in sex, as well as an increase in body fat and a decrease in muscle mass and bone density. While those side effects were significant, and I was experiencing many of them, they didn't address why I came to tears more easily and more often.

I kept digging until I found an article on the American Psychological Association website that addressed the psychology of tears and asked the question, "Why does one person get choked up over a Hallmark commercial, while another sheds tears only for the death of a loved one?" The article pointed out that studies over the years and across the world have found that women cry more than men. While that was no surprise, the article went on to suggest that there may be a biological reason for this difference: prolactin, a hormone found in higher levels in women, may promote crying, while testosterone in men may inhibit it.

I also found articles that reported how some men undergoing hormone therapy for prostate cancer cried more often. Learning that other men in treatment shed tears reduced my embarrassment.

Embarrassed or not, I was glad I cried with Mary. Sharing that tearful moment during the veteran's funeral and hoping for other emotional moments was, to my testosterone-lacking self, a positive side effect of hormone therapy. Crying was a form of intimacy that brought us closer as we supported each other. That closeness felt even more important with the loss of sexual intimacy.

I experienced another instance of crying, this time triggered by a very different situation. I was going to install a new controller to improve our internet service. Having installed other devices before, I expected the process to be easy.

I began first thing in the morning, my best mental time of day. The only physical part of the job was plugging the controller in and placing it near various windows to see where it received the best cell signal. Once I found the right spot, I placed the controller there and took a seat. Then came all the button pushing on the controller's phone app as I tried to connect our phones, computers, and other gadgets. I made connections, but not without problems. My frustration was a slow burn: I mumbled and cursed softly.

The situation escalated as I struggled to connect the last gadget. Try as I might, I couldn't make that connection. To make matters worse, I kept pushing the same buttons in the same order, while somehow expecting a different result. *Isn't that one definition of insanity?* I thought, but I didn't stop the pushing. My mumbling grew louder and more frequent. When I shouted some curse words, Mary yelled from the other room, "Do you need some help?" My inner high achiever lied and said that I didn't. More button pushing, more failure, more cursing. I stood and felt like throwing my phone through the dining room window. Instead, I gave up and yelled, "Yeah, I need some help."

Mary came out, I showed her what I had done, handed her the phone, and wished her luck. I stood by her shoulder, watched her push buttons without success, and felt my frustration rising further. But Mary stayed calm, persisted, and figured out the needed step. The final gadget was connected.

She looked at me, handed me the phone, and said, "There, we did it."

I was surprised to feel tears forming. She saw this and hugged me. I put my head on her shoulder and began to cry. "Let it go. Let it go," she whispered. I sobbed.

When I could finally speak, I thanked Mary for her support and wondered why this process had been so frustrating. I had installed other internet devices, and while there had been problems, I had never cried or wanted to throw my phone through a window. Could that extreme frustration be another side effect of low testosterone?

I headed online again and found a paper published in the American Cancer Society Journals that reviewed how studies found many men with prostate cancer felt more emotionally responsive during hormone therapy when their testosterone levels were low. Some men reported feeling more sensitive or sentimental, while others felt more irritable and angry.

I was surprised to read that the most marked change was the experience of becoming more spontaneously tearful, particularly in situations that previously would not produce tears, which fit with my crying while watching the veteran's funeral and struggling with the gadget.

The paper reported that some men found this tearfulness confusing and difficult to understand, while others, like me, felt embarrassed. The researchers concluded that how men perceived this increase in emotionality and whether or not they accepted it may influence how well they adapt to hormone therapy and prostate cancer.

I was relieved to find those studies that helped me put my emotional moments into perspective. I wasn't going crazy. I was struggling with another side effect of hormone therapy.

Of course, therapy would not last forever; it would end in less than twelve months. Then, my testosterone could rise again, though that was not guaranteed because of my age. Would more testosterone reduce my willingness to shed a tear over something as "minor" as a sad scene on TV? Would more testosterone make me less vulnerable to tears of frustration? Or would these changes in how I felt and dealt with emotions be permanent?

I looked forward to answering those questions.

CHAPTER 37

Tale of Two Brothers

My BROTHER—WHO IS FOUR YEARS OLDER—WAS DIAGNOSED with prostate cancer a couple of years before me. His cancer was not very aggressive, and he is on active surveillance. My aggressive cancer called for immediate treatment. This situation brought up two questions. Was it coincidental or hereditary that two brothers had prostate cancer? Why would one brother's cancer be more aggressive? Seeking to answer those questions led me to a tale of two brothers.

First, I started clicking around online to see whether prostate cancer can be hereditary. I found that both the National Cancer Institute and the American Cancer Society discussed hereditary factors in prostate cancer. While most prostate cancer is not hereditary, some is. I was struck by this statement on the ACS website: "Having a father or brother with prostate cancer more than doubles a man's risk of developing this disease. (The risk is higher for men who have a brother with the disease than for those who have a father with it.)"

I don't know whether our father was ever diagnosed with prostate cancer, and genetically gifted my brother and me. He was an alcoholic who also smoked far too many cigarettes all his life. He died from illnesses related to both harmful habits. Hereditary or coincidental, there's no doubt that my brother and I both have prostate cancer. But why are our cancers so different in their aggressiveness?

I sat back and pondered that question, considering our bodies and lifestyles. I concluded that while my brother and I were different in several ways, one distinction could be critical: my lifelong sugar addiction.

I had researched the connection between sugar and prostate cancer many months ago when Mary and I began changing our diet. I had found a study that showed increased consumption of sugars from sugar-sweetened beverages, such as soda, was linked with an increased risk of prostate cancer for men, like me, who were in the highest quartile of sugar consumption. I eliminated all added sugar from my diet, while still consuming fruits and vegetables that contain natural sugars.

As I delved into the topic again, I learned that whether sugar, natural or added, is harmful depends on how quickly it is absorbed. The American Heart Association states on its website: "…your body spends more time digesting an apple because of the fiber content, so the natural sugar absorbs more slowly. Conversely, the added sugar in soda arrives all at once in your system like a sugar bomb." That bomb starts a process that actually nurtures prostate cancer cells. I had sugar-bombed my body every day for decades.

An article on the Prostate Cancer Foundation website supported the importance of diet and quotes one researcher as saying: "The more we learn about cancer metabolism, we are understanding that cancers are addicted to particular things. For many cancers, that thing is sugar." The article concludes: "One day, in addition to surgery, radiation, hormonal therapy, or other treatments for prostate cancer, patients will be prescribed a precision diet to make the treatment more successful."

With sugar on my mind—but still not in the coffee I was sipping—I called my brother. First, I summarized the connection between sugar and prostate cancer. Then I described my sugar-addicted intake—how I used to consistently consume more than three times the current American Heart Association's sugar recommendation for men. He listened in silence, and when I stopped, he whistled softly and said, "My God, Rick, that's a lot of sugar."

I agreed and asked him to describe his sugar consumption.

"Everything you just mentioned," he said, "I didn't do and still don't do." Further questioning confirmed he had no sugar addiction and only a small intake of added sugar.

Ending the call, I sat there, phone in hand, considering this tale of two brothers. Each may have had a hereditary risk of developing prostate cancer. One brother was not a sugar addict and consumed little added sugar each day.

He did not spike his blood sugar and feed his prostate cancer cells. Instead, his cancer cells had to live in a sugar-starved environment; they survived but multiplied less. Finally, that brother's PSA and a biopsy revealed those slow-growing cancer cells. However, they were not well-fed, not overly aggressive, and he was under active surveillance.

The other brother was a sugar addict, oblivious to sugar-bombing his cancer cells with repeated sweet treats. Every day, after multiple blood sugar spikes, his prostate cancer cells feasted. Month after month, year after year, decade after decade, he created a nourishing environment for those little killers. Finally, after fifty years of sugar addiction, his high PSA and a biopsy revealed the presence of an aggressive prostate cancer that required immediate hormone therapy and radiation.

After again immersing myself in the topic of sugar and prostate cancer, I think this tale of two brothers—this connection between sugar intake and prostate cancer—is possible. However, I'm not a scientist or doctor. I'm a guy with regrets and wishes. I regret my sugar addiction and wish I had opened my eyes and closed my mouth to that dangerous habit long ago. But I can't erase that mistake.

What I can do is minimize its impact by focusing every day on my diet and avoiding added sugar. I can become addicted to starving those cancer cells that I fed for so many years.

CHAPTER 38

Connecting

THREE MONTHS AGO, I TOLD MYSELF I SHOULD AND WOULD start building deeper relationships with men friends to strengthen my cancer-fighting support system. But I made little effort to do so. Until I read a *Psychology Today* article by Marisa G. Franco, Ph.D., a psychologist and friendship expert, who had interviewed Billy Baker, the author of *We Need to Hang Out: A Memoir of Making Friends.*

Baker, at the age of forty, had, like many other men, settled into a busy career and active family life. When he accepted an assignment to write an article about today's loneliness epidemic, he was surprised to find that about fifty million Americans over the age of forty-five, especially men, suffer from chronic loneliness. Surprise turned to shock when he realized he met the criteria for inclusion in the lonely cohort. To understand this epidemic and what could be done to overcome loneliness, he read studies and consulted with sociologists, psychologists, and experts on friendship. His findings inspired him to rejuvenate lost friendships and write the book.

In her article, Franco summarized three high points of her interview with Baker: First, to make friends, "men likely need to disrupt ideas about masculinity. This includes being vulnerable and showing care." Next, while spouse and family relationships are important, "so is friendship. Men can make friendship a priority by checking in and making plans with friends." Finally, making those regular plans "gives men an excuse to meet up and build friendship."

Those three points resonated with me. I wanted to be more vulnerable and caring. I wanted to make friendship a priority. I wanted to build friendships with men. What was I waiting for?

The article helped me push myself to schedule phone calls with three men. Time—in some cases, years—had passed since I had talked at length or in depth with them. My past connection with each had centered around sharing a specific activity; sharing feelings had taken second place. There was a man whom I had connected with during my wolf advocacy days. Another man had been my adventure partner during hundreds of miles of self-supported bicycle touring across the West. Finally, there was a fellow writer with whom I had experienced the joys and struggles of writing.

How, I wondered, would those calls go? I was sure each man had changed over time, just as I had. I was once a full-time advocate, an active adventurer, and a productive writer. Since being diagnosed with prostate cancer, I had stepped away from advocating. I adventured less. I had turned writing into journaling and visiting my paper therapist.

I longed to explore how such changes fit into being a man, especially an aging man. Were my friends experiencing these or other issues? How did they feel about them? Were they suffering from health issues? How did they feel about that?

Oh, come on, Rick, my inner critic shouted, *these are phone calls with old friends, not some seminar you're leading. Mellow out!*

But should I? It's so easy to stay on the surface. It's so challenging, as Franco noted, to explore and share feelings. But sharing was what I sought. I needed to be honest with each man about that. I would respect whatever each decided regarding connecting on a deeper level.

The feelings I wanted to share were not unusual. A psychologist and pioneer in the study of emotions, Paul Ekman, identifies seven universal emotions: fear, surprise, anger, sadness, enjoyment, disgust, and contempt. Battling cancer led me to experience most of them. I was surprised and angry to find cancer inside me. I feared how cancer could change my life. I was sad to face my mortality again. Those feelings were somewhat offset by the enjoyment of hiking, skiing, canoeing, and bicycling in wild lands and near wildlife.

But dealing with cancer had exposed a disturbing lack: I had many emotions inside me, but few men to share them with. And I had created this problem.

When we lived in Oregon, I helped organize those men's retreats. When I attended, I shared deeply with other men. However, I left those retreats and the sharing that occurred when we moved to Montana.

In Gardiner, I chose to focus instead on learning about the ecosystem and wildlife, particularly wolves and bison. I explored Yellowstone and the surrounding national forest with men I wanted to become friends with. Most were long-time residents of Gardiner, and all were knowledgeable about the local ecosystem. I enjoyed listening to what they had learned about the wild land and wildlife around us.

Over the years of field time with those men, I learned a great deal that helped me advocate, and I developed solid friendships. But they were not based on deep personal sharing. If we discussed feelings, it was usually how much awe we felt while watching wildlife or how much we loved living in such a wild and wonder-filled place.

I'll never forget, for example, the day we watched a hungry lone wolf encounter a tempting lone bison. Watching the much-smaller predator approach its possible prey and seeing the bison chase the wolf away opened my eyes to the necessity of wolves hunting in packs. Working together, wolves increase their chances of survival.

Thinking about how wolves made their lives better by hunting in packs, I wondered if I could improve my life by forming a pack of male friends. I certainly craved sharing on a deeper level, in different ways, with different men. Was this another side effect of low testosterone? Had facing my mortality brought this situation to a head? Was aging the culprit? It could be a combination of all three.

For whatever reason, I was determined to make the scheduled phone calls and try to reconnect with those three men. When each asked, "How are you doing?" I would not spend much time on the physical part of this cancer journey. I would dive into the emotional side and look for what I needed. My heart sought this shared connection; my mind was unsure why. I would listen to my heart.

After several calls with the three men friends, I was pleased to find I was not alone. Two of the men said they enjoyed our sharing and had few male friends with whom to share deeply. We were discovering ways to help ourselves go deeper, and I wanted to find more. This would be my next learning on this life-affirming journey: connecting and sharing on a deeper level. I wanted to spend my last years, however many there may be, in a quality life with some men knowing my heart and me knowing theirs.

CHAPTER 39

Back to the Battle

Mary and I were on vacation, visiting family and friends in Oregon and Washington. More than seven months into treatment, I had gladly left behind the research and journaling. I had driven away from the daily wondering and worrying about my prostate cancer and my future. I had cruised into being present with loved ones. What a joy!

Mary and I were lounging on the deck of our room on the third floor of an oceanfront hotel in Newport, Oregon. We had a fine view of the Pacific Ocean's incoming tide, a view we had often enjoyed during our many years living in Oregon. After moving to Montana, we missed being near the ocean and jumped at every chance to revisit.

As I watched and listened to the waves breaking, I felt relaxed, relieved to have focused on something other than cancer for three whole weeks. But as the time approached to tackle the long, snowy drive home to Montana, I could feel myself slipping back into battle mode. My R&R, my rest and relaxation, was coming to an end. I would soon return to the front lines in this fight against that deadly adversary within.

When first diagnosed, I had viewed that enemy as an invader. But I was wrong. Those prostate cancer cells didn't invade my body; they began life as my healthy cells. Until something went terribly wrong: they lost their ability to control their reproduction. They ran rampant, using my body's helpful processes against me. They drew strength from my testosterone, as I do. They gained energy from blood sugar spikes, as I do. Without treatment and left to their own devices, these once-healthy cells that had somehow become immortal would slowly spread to other parts of my body and eventually kill me, the host that sustains them. But I had refused to let those tough little buggers that had survived weeks of radiation shots and months of starvation from hormone therapy win without a fight.

Sitting on that deck, enjoying the endless ocean's sight, sound, and scent, I felt energized and ready to DARE to fight treatment side effects and those surviving cancer cells. I was prepared to recommit with my body, mind, and heart to this battle.

A few weeks later, back home, I experienced a new front in the battle when my medical records app notified me that my recent blood work results were available. I reviewed the data and identified several concerns and questions to discuss with the oncologist. I sent him a message requesting a phone call. Based on previous experience, I expected a nurse would answer first and then have him call me within a day or so.

But not this time: it took seven long days of messaging back and forth with the nurse to get the oncologist to call. Even worse, in her third message, the nurse said I should first follow up with my primary care physician regarding my concerns about the blood work. I countered that before I bothered my primary care physician, I wanted to speak with the oncologist. She said she would have him call me.

While waiting for the call, I conducted additional research to address my questions and concerns. I wanted to have an intelligent and satisfying discussion with the doctor. I wanted to engage in shared decision-making, a process in which healthcare providers collaborate with patients to make informed decisions about appropriate treatment. Shared decision-making uses the best available evidence, clinical expertise, along with the patient's values, preferences, and circumstances to arrive at treatment decisions. My research helped me understand the treatment options and identify my preferences.

Five days later, after receiving no call, I messaged the nurse again. In addition to feeling frustrated, I was surprised. In the nine months I had been dealing with my Cancer Center medical team, that was the first time I experienced such a delay.

Finally, the oncologist called, and we engaged in shared decision-making. We discussed my questions and concerns about the blood work. I was glad I had spent the time and energy to educate myself; I understood what he was saying to me. And I asked questions that made him stop and think and even reconsider. At the conclusion of our call, I summarized that, based on his comments and my research findings, I did not need to be concerned with the changes in the blood work. I did not need to involve my primary care doctor. The oncologist agreed.

Seven days of back-and-forth messaging provided a good example of another front in this battle: sometimes, patients must invest the time and energy in advocating for themselves. I was glad I had educated myself, persisted, engaged in shared decision-making, and kept asking questions until I had answers that did not raise more questions.

CHAPTER 40

Stuck in the Middle

Silent and resting, I sat by the picture window in the dining room, watching the sun descend toward the summit of nearby Sepulcher Mountain. The sunlit pattern on Sepulcher's flank, created by bright snow and dark conifers, resembled the face of a river otter with a large dark nose, two dark eyes, and some dark lines of conifers defining the top of the head. The rumpled hills that began at Sepulcher's base and continued down to the Yellowstone River were losing their snow cover as spring slowly unfolded.

Near our picture window, some robins drank from a partially thawed bird bath. An energetic robin hopped and hunted in the flower bed below the window. Recently, Mary had pulled from that bed the roots and skeletons of last year's giant sunflowers, exposing many insects that had been hidden beneath the surface. The robin was dining on those that had not dug back to safety. Beyond the flower bed, the snow-free lawn was a blend of yellow and light green grass freckled with dried brown aspen leaves that had emerged from a deep freeze beneath winter's snow. Shrubs in the yard were sprouting leaves; blossoms should not be far behind.

Yesterday morning, like that industrious robin, Mary and I hopped into a flurry of spring activity. We officially called winter over and ended the ski season. We hung our skis and poles, stored our snow tires, and removed our car-top cargo carrier. She raked up dead leaves, and I got the mower ready for another season. Afterward, I came inside to fix lunch and take a much-needed nap. I felt troubled that, as I entered my eighth month of hormone therapy, napping seemed more essential than ever. And I was slower to climb out of bed afterward.

Yesterday evening, as Mary and I discussed our joy in watching spring arrive and our excitement about working together in the yard as the days grew longer and warmer, I admitted to her my fear that I might not have the energy to be as much help as I had in the past.

She looked puzzled and asked, "Why's that?"

"I've had to talk myself into tackling my two strength routines these last few weeks. Worse yet, after a recent workout, I fixed myself a protein smoothie, sank into this chair, read for a few minutes, and nodded off into my second nap of the day. And when I awoke, my energy never materialized. I walked around, sighing and muttering, "It's official; I'm feeling more fatigued."

Having shared my struggles with exercise, I pushed myself to admit to her how I was struggling to meet other

DARE targets. With diet, I had slacked off on eating as many cancer-fighting foods as possible. With rest, I was less consistent with taking afternoon naps and paid for that later in the day. With attitude, I found myself wondering, *Is all this worth it?*

"It's crazy," I concluded. "I'm wrestling with these goals, and I'm still two weeks away from the halfway point in hormone therapy."

Mary nodded, saying, "I've struggled at midpoints, too, especially with long-term projects."

"Huh, so have I," I said, surprised that I hadn't thought about that. "And there's no doubt that eighteen months of hormone therapy is long-term."

A couple of days later, while sipping my morning coffee, I mulled over the concept of the midpoint. Is there research supporting our observations about midpoint struggles? If so, what could I learn that would help me? I went online looking for scholarly articles.

I located an eleven-year-old study cited numerous times and appropriately titled "Stuck in the Middle: The Psychophysics of Goal Pursuit." The researchers found that in the middle, when the starting and end points are equidistant, motivation fades, and a person may give up on reaching the end goal and become stuck. They also found that motivation can increase as the end comes into sight. The researchers wrote that to avoid being stuck, "Early in your pursuit of your goal, look backward at what you have achieved; toward the end, look forward."

I also found sources on setting goals. One study reported that only 8% of people who set New Year's resolutions achieved them. When researchers examined how these achievers succeeded, they found that setting specific and challenging goals helped individuals perform better. I wondered if my overarching goal of making my body a hostile environment for prostate cancer cells and a haven for healthy cells was too vague and was, in fact, part of the problem.

Perhaps I needed to break that big goal into smaller, more manageable chunks. Our DARE approach provided a helpful framework for doing that. During each upcoming month, I would conduct a one-week food check to ensure my diet included cancer-fighting foods each day. I would also complete a one-week sleep check to ensure my sleep provided my body with the necessary rest and restorative deep sleep. I would attend two cancer-related webinars to help maintain a positive attitude. And, finally, I would exercise five times a week, including strength and aerobic sessions.

I would review my results weekly and at the end of each month. If I met those new specific objectives, I should feel rewarded and motivated to continue using the approach in the upcoming weeks.

I ended the day with a vision of staying motivated, unstuck, and on track one week at a time. I would not be stuck in the middle.

CHAPTER 41

On the Edge

I PARKED THE CAR, AND MARY AND I SLUNG OUR PACKS, grabbed our hiking poles, and started the first hike of spring. I was excited about spending a day letting nature help me recover from the side effects of nine months of treatment. At the trailhead, we stopped and stared at the trail: a snowy slash through green sage. Though we had hiked this route several times, this would be our first time over what looked like crusty old snow.

We stepped up onto the snowy trail and began what I call crust-creeping, treading across the crust ever so gently, hoping not to break through. Within a few steps, my stationary foot slid sideways on the snowy crust as I lifted my other foot into the air. I almost fell into the sage, but jamming my hiking poles into the snow saved me.

After a few more slippery steps, we agreed to leave the slick trail and take our chances in the sage, where the snow was either light or had already melted. As we climbed a steep slope, we detoured around snow patches.

Occasionally, we chose crust-creeping as the shortest route. A couple of times, the crust broke, our feet sank, and the snow reached calf or knee height, slipping into our boots and chilling our feet.

But we kept going, stopping occasionally to admire the view of snow-covered mountains. We listened to the nearby waterfall; rushing snowmelt had filled the creek, which roared over the edge. Two mountain bluebirds, a male and a female, flew by, chirping at one another. He had likely shown her his nest, and she had accepted it and him. Now, they were flying, flirting, and feeding, waiting for eggs to arrive.

Smiling at the energy of the bluebirds, I decided to make this hike a strength workout as well as an aerobic one. I used my poles to help pull me up the steep slope, feeling my arms, chest, and core muscles strain. My breathing grew heavy. My heart pumped. I felt energized.

We soon reached the part of the hike where we had to navigate up and down two wide gullies. Descending the first gully required more crust-creeping. Every time I broke through, I had to fight being toppled as my upper body continued forward while my feet stuck in knee-deep snow. This step-by-step struggle tired me and killed my energy. We found a snow-free bison trail at the bottom of the gully and used it to climb up and out. I silently thanked our four-legged friends.

As we climbed into and out of the second gully, I recalled that we would soon reach a cliff and an awe-inspiring view from a trail that winds for a couple more miles along the edge of this flat mountaintop. But as I huffed out of the forested gully, my thoughts were conflicted: *What an incredible hike! When are we going to stop?*

While thoughts like those often occurred around lunchtime or toward the end of a longer hike, we had only hiked a mile, and lunchtime was at least an hour away. I felt uneasy about flagging so soon. I kept my mouth shut and didn't tell Mary how I felt.

Leaving the gully, we stepped out of the forest and into that eye-popping viewscape. But even with a thrilling view, my energy sagged with each step. Moments later, I gave in when we reached a viewpoint on the cliff's edge. I threw my pack to the ground, pulled out my lunch and water, chose a stone—lichen-covered and rainbow-colored—as a seat, and released a long, tired breath.

Mary stood a few feet away as I ripped into my sandwich and an early lunch. I watched her gaze longingly at the next higher viewpoint.

"If you want to keep going," I muttered with my mouth full, "that's fine with me."

"Yeah, I think I'd like that," she replied with a smile.

Swallowing, I said clearly, "Go for it. I'll sit here and watch. Don't let me hold you back. I'm just beat."

"Maybe you should take a nap."

"Maybe."

As Mary progressed along the cliffside trail, she was hidden when passing through stands of conifers. When she reached a viewpoint and emerged into full view, she was a lone hiker on a promontory framed by green conifers, a blue sky, and a snow-capped mountain backdrop. I put down my sandwich, dug out my camera, and snapped photo after photo.

Putting the camera away, I leaned forward to study the sheer red cliff at my feet and the large boulders clustered far below at its base. As I looked down, a thought popped into my head: *This would be a good place to jump if I wanted to end it all.*

Shocked, I shook my head, leaned back, and wondered, *Where the hell did that come from?*

Then: *Well, what do I do with it?* I could try to ignore and deny. But as I looked away from the cliff and toward distant Electric Peak, that mountain we admire from our dining room window, I recalled my commitment to not ignore my thoughts and feelings—no matter how distressing they might be—as I fought cancer.

Alright, I won't deny the thought, but why think like that? I pondered this question as I watched a raven soar below me. As the bird flew away, I recalled a long and recent phone conversation with a friend whose prostate cancer had spread after he underwent the same treatment I was going through. He understood that with the spread, there was no cure, only more treatment to relieve symptoms and give him more time. He told me that after suffering several pain-filled years, he had recently decided that he would accept no more treatment. He was ready to go. *Ah, he was prepared to jump off his figurative cliff.*

If, after my treatment ends, my cancer spreads, and I tire of fighting and suffering, there could be a cliff for me. As troubling and disconcerting as that thought felt while surrounded by nature's wonders, I felt good to have acknowledged, faced, and accepted it.

As I looked across the chasm at Mary, standing at yet another viewpoint, I had another life-affirming thought. I realized that in places like this, with her, was where I wanted to be for as long as possible. So be it if treatment-caused fatigue cuts my hikes in half. I would respect my body's limitations, but I would keep moving. Every minute in this wonderland could help me feel stronger, more present, and more alive. And better able to accept any end that lies ahead on this journey into the wilds of prostate cancer.

CHAPTER 42

A Peak a Week

SINCE THAT SPRING HIKE THREE MONTHS AGO, STRUGGLING with crusty snow and fatigue and scaring myself on that cliff, I have hiked regularly with Mary, mostly on flat or rolling terrain. But as summer finally melted the snow from the mountains around us, the peaks called.

Hiking to summits was one of the reasons we chose to leave Oregon and move to Gardiner, a tiny town surrounded by abundant mountains with official or social trails to their peaks. Summer was the time to summit, sit, stare at wild views, and feel fortunate to live in such a place.

I missed those high moments last summer after receiving my cancer diagnosis on the summer solstice. Medical appointments and treatment visits ate up my time. The reality of battling cancer took a heavy emotional toll. The side effects of radiation treatments and months of hormone therapy sapped my energy and desire to hike. With all those cancer-related physical and emotional challenges filling the summer, I reached the summit of only one peak — a new low for me.

In the eleven months since treatment began, I've dealt with most, but not all, of the emotional challenges. Physically, the radiation side effects were behind me, and I was managing the hormone therapy side effects. I've found that more time passes between my intense visits to my paper therapist. And I've found that I am ready, willing, and mostly able to commit to a peak a week for the summer.

Although I began by carefully choosing peaks with shorter hikes and less elevation gain that would challenge but not overwhelm me, I still encountered difficulties. My leg muscles felt weak, making climbing steep slopes more difficult. Loss of muscle mass, a side effect of long-term hormone therapy, was probably the culprit. I also felt more fatigued, which reduced my endurance. That change was likely due to my low testosterone level, another side-effect of hormone therapy. With less strength and more fatigue, I often brought up the rear instead of being further forward in the pack of friends that Mary and I sometimes hike with.

After struggling up and down several peaks, I realized I needed to change my attitude to help me cope. I needed to accept that stopping more often to catch my breath and recharge was not all bad. The breaks offered opportunities to be present, observe, and photograph.

Sometimes, I got lost in the views of mountains that seemed to stretch forever. Sometimes, I photographed my healthier hiking partners as they climbed away from me. Sometimes, I was captivated by the colorful wildflowers in full bloom; some waved in the breeze, others clung to the ground. Sometimes, I was thankful to spot wildlife, the winged and four-legged friends that live or visit at higher elevations.

Ever so slowly, I convinced my inner high achiever to accept the logical conclusion of that new attitude: I didn't need to reach every summit; I was out there for the joy of being in nature with my friends.

One day, after a particularly challenging peak, when I was sitting at home resting, recovering, and rebuilding, I went online seeking information on how others coped with the physical challenges brought on by cancer and treatment. I found a recent study entitled "Nature-Based Interventions and Exposure among Cancer Survivors: A Scoping Review."

The study analyzed the scientific literature on nature-based interventions, which include viewing nature, being surrounded by nature, and engaging with nature. (My struggling up a peak a week included all three.) While such interventions have been shown to positively affect the physical, psychological, social, and spiritual health of the larger population, this review specifically examined the impact of nature-based interventions on cancer survivors.

The review found twelve studies describing 2,786 cancer survivors with multiple types and stages of cancer. The studies showed that nature-based interventions had a positive impact on the quality of life, physical activity, inflammation, immune system function, stress, anxiety, and blood pressure in cancer survivors. Time in nature also improved sleep and decreased depression, confusion, fatigue, and pain. Participants in the studies reported that nature was the most important resource in coping with cancer.

The review concluded that nature-based interventions were beneficial for cancer survivors who participated in them during diagnosis and treatment. Furthermore, nature opportunities and their benefits could also be purposefully delivered to more cancer patients. In fact, using nature to help needs to be "explored further and safely implemented to support the overall health and well-being of cancer survivors."

The research convinced me that I did not need to summit every peak. Instead, I should focus on viewing, being surrounded by, and engaging with nature on every hike, regardless of how high I climb. Time in nature, not just time on the peak, will help me fight cancer.

CHAPTER 43

The New Normal

AFTER SIXTEEN MONTHS, I WAS FINALLY CLOSING IN ON the end of medical treatment. I was no longer stuck in the middle. I was looking forward to my final treatment appointment in just two months. Three months after that, I would attend my first follow-up appointment. By then, the hormone that was injected into my body during hormone therapy to stop testosterone production should be out of my body. If so, my testosterone levels should increase, unless my age creates a problem. As the levels increase, I should experience a gradual decline in the side effects of low testosterone and enter a new normal.

I first thought about this new normal after a recent conversation with a friend whose prostate cancer had spread. He was deep in the throes of more treatment: two medications that reduced testosterone plus sessions of chemotherapy with a drug that kills cancer cells as well as healthy cells. As he described his significant side effects, I realized that my moderating side effects had helped me enter that new normal.

The time in nature last summer, struggling to hike a peak a week, had brought healing and joy, whether I reached summits or not. As fall faded, I still fought fatigue, but the level had been decreasing. Honestly, the current fatigue could be more related to my exercise regimen and age than hormone therapy. My gastrointestinal issues, my GIs, had also gone away since my bladder and rectum had calmed down after radiation ended almost a year ago.

When my friend shared how his life was now filled with stress, I remembered how stressful my first few months after diagnosis had been. I was overloaded with fear, anxiety, and uncertainty as I faced cancer, treatment, and mortality. But facing mortality had become less prevalent. I still accepted the threat of my cancer spreading and leading to more troubling treatment and even death. After all, my oncologist had given me a fifty percent chance of a recurrence; I would be foolish not to focus on that threat. Its presence motivated me to keep up the fight.

But most days, I enjoyed my relatively stress-free time with Mary, family, and friends, especially in nature. I told Mary about my entering a new normal and even revealed that I was wondering whether we might travel next spring, summer, or fall. I told her how happy I was to be enjoying the present and imagining a future.

That was quite different than when I began the months of the one-two punch of hormone therapy and radiation. Then, treatment, side effects, and the likelihood of success were all I thought about as I grieved having cancer. I didn't consider taking any trips; my GIs kept me close to the bathroom. I didn't think much about the future; I wasn't sure I had a future. Instead, I was consumed by dealing with my grief through denial, anger, and bargaining, three of the five stages of grief described by psychiatrist Kübler-Ross.

Luckily, I didn't dip into depression, another stage. Instead, when I journaled each morning and found myself sounding or feeling depressed, I did as I had promised to do: I acknowledged those feelings, explored them, and made them my own. Having done that, I took steps that could change my outlook: Go for an aerobic walk. Share with a friend. Focus on the positive and hopeful.

Just weeks ago, I finally arrived at acceptance, the remaining stage of grief, when I found myself journaling: *This is how it is right now. I've got cancer, but I also have a life to live. Get on with it.* I accepted my cancer, my treatment, and the lifestyle changes caused by both. I also accepted that the future could change for the worse. If it did, I could adapt and respond, prepare and persist. Since my diagnosis, I have learned how to fight cancer. Though I hesitated to write this, I even felt hopeful that we had won this battle. I was almost ready to call myself a cancer survivor. At the very least, we had achieved a ceasefire.

But this war would never end. Though radiation and hormone therapy brought on struggles, my oncologist had warned me that the burning and starving would probably not kill all the microscopic cancer cells. Given that, I decided to be vigilant every day to help my body beat those tough little survivors and avoid the risk of a recurrence.

I could do that if I stayed committed to DARE, which would soon become my first line of defense once conventional medical treatment ended. Our diet was filled with tasty cancer-fighting foods. Sufficient rest allowed my body, mind, and heart to recover each night. Consistent exercise helped my body rebuild. A positive and hopeful attitude helped me focus and commit to the other components.

In the new normal, diet, attitude, rest, exercise, and time in nature had become my personal, proactive, and life-affirming prescription for keeping cancer at bay.

CHAPTER 44

Facing Fear, Feeling Hope

WHEN THE WEBINAR ENDED, I SIGHED, SHUT DOWN THE computer, and shuffled to the kitchen. Turning a corner, I saw Mary standing at the stove, stirring colorful sautéed vegetables. I stopped, leaned against a counter, and said nothing.

Mary put down her spoon and studied my face. "Are you alright?" she asked.

I wondered if I should tell her what I was feeling, given that just three weeks ago, I had shared with her that reassuring sense of a new normal. Would this roller coaster never end? But I needed to say the words. "I'm scared," I grumbled.

We closed the gap between us and hugged. Tears came to my eyes as I whispered, "Really scared." I felt her warmth and strength as she reminded me again, "Rick, you're going to get through this. We're going to get through this."

We held the hug a moment longer, and then she returned to cooking. As she worked, I explained how the evening's webinar on metastatic prostate cancer had tapped into a haunting fear, as the chief medical officer of the Prostate Cancer Foundation interviewed two cancer specialists.

At one point, the trio discussed treatment when prostate cancer cells spread to other parts of the body and become advanced prostate cancer. While they talked, a slide titled "Treatment Landscape for Advanced Prostate Cancer" appeared on the screen. Across the center of the slide was a jagged red line that formed the outline of a row of three mountain peaks. Below the red mountains was a straight blue line indicating a time frame of ten to twenty years. Along the red peaks were arrows identifying points where specific treatments were appropriate. Past the last peak and last treatment, the red line ended at one word: Death. That was my haunting fear: if my cancer spread to other parts of my body, there would be no cure.

While they calmly discussed various treatments, I stared at the slide and that one scary word. But for the doctors, the slide provided a reason to be grateful: treatment had improved as technology had advanced. And, of course, they were right. The advances and new treatments were incredible and could help them reach their stated goal: fighting metastatic prostate cancer while maintaining a good quality of life.

"That's exactly what we're looking for, more quality years," Mary said.

I nodded and said nothing as I again pictured that word at the end of the jagged red treatment line.

Mary seemed to read my mind as she said, "We're all going to die, Rick. It's just a matter of when and how." She tapped her chest and said, "Maybe my heart will give out." She pointed at me, "Maybe it's cancer for you. Or maybe we take a fall while hiking on a mountainside and plummet to our end. Who knows when or how? What really matters is what we do every day to fight your cancer."

I sniffled and said, "You're right. It's what we do every day."

As Mary returned to dinner prep, I smiled, pointed to the stove, and added, "And the doctors did mention how important diet is."

"We're doing the right things," Mary said, grinning and pointing to the quinoa, tofu, and colorful veggies in the saucepan.

"They also mentioned the importance of exercise. And I had a great walk today along the Yellowstone River. I pushed myself, felt strong, glad to be alive."

Mary pulled me into another hug and whispered, "And I'm glad you're alive. So far, the treatment is working. You just have a couple more months, and then you get your body back again. You can beat this. We can beat this."

I pulled my head back so I could look at her. The smile on her confident face and the love in her eyes obliterated the image of that red line and scary word.

The next day, after I journaled and shared my thoughts with my paper therapist about my tears and fears in the kitchen, I turned back to the notes I had scribbled in my journal during the troubling webinar. I had jotted down how one doctor had emphasized that the majority of men with localized prostate cancer like mine won't die from the cancer. And if the cancer spreads, the doctors have options. They would treat the whole patient, emphasizing lifestyle changes, general health, diet, and exercise. They would use smarter, more targeted treatments to better personalize the therapy. They would prolong life, improve symptoms, and delay the disease so that, in the future, men with advanced prostate cancer could live longer and better.

In those notes, I found reasons to be optimistic. But first, I had to own my powerful fear and admit it to Mary and my paper therapist. Facing fear allowed me to feel hope.

CHAPTER 45

Determined

MARY AND I WILL ATTEND MY FINAL TREATMENT APPOINT-ment in a few days. I was amazed that almost eighteen months had gone by since that first hormone therapy injection. But it had, and we could see the end of treatment and the beginning of follow-up. We wanted to celebrate that transition with a ski. But the snow had been light so far this winter, and we were not sure the trail we wanted — one of our favorites in Yellowstone — would be skiable. But, as we are fond of saying when wondering about the conditions for a hike or ski, "You never know till you get to the trailhead."

That statement also applied to this trip into the wilds of cancer, since I envisioned the upcoming first follow-up appointment as the trailhead of the next leg of the journey. We wouldn't know the challenges the new trail would present until we met with the doctor and reviewed the day's blood work. Just like we wanted to see good snow on the ski trail, we wanted to see a good PSA that would indicate few — if any — prostate cancer cells were active in my body. We also longed to see an increase in my testosterone level. More testosterone would mean fewer side effects, less fatigue, and I wanted both on this new trail.

We decided to take our chances and make the long drive to the favorite ski trail. When Mary parked the car in the small, empty lot at the trailhead, the temperature was barely above zero. Luckily, the trail was covered with a few inches of snow and a skier-broken track. We cheered, bumped fists, and pushed off. Let the celebration begin!

A chilly celebration, for sure. As I wiggled my fingers and thumbs constantly while grasping my ski poles, Mary yelled from behind me, "My fingers are freezing!"

"Mine too!" I picked up my pace, hoping to warm my blood and get it flowing to my fingers.

"But I'm so glad to be out here," Mary said.

We had been inside for the last three days as temperatures fell to as low as minus twenty-eight, with daytime highs, like today's, barely above zero. Looking around at Yellowstone's wild beauty, I felt a slight burn as my lungs drew in frigid air. But I smiled, happy to be in nature and soon out of treatment.

After about a mile of climbing, the celebration abruptly ended. My vision went haywire. The light dimmed. The snow, bright white a moment ago, faded to gray. The snow-flocked trees along the trail slipped out of focus. I wobbled. Felt like I was out of my body.

Scared, I slowed and stopped. My vision began to return, but my whole body started tingling. Not shivering; tingling. I looked around, wondering if this was where I would pass out and fall into the snow. What would Mary do? Hoping to avoid a crisis, I drove my poles into the snow, leaned on them, and told myself to breathe, relax, breathe, relax.

I sensed Mary arriving on my left. While it's not unusual for one of us to stop to adjust gear, look around, or take a photograph, this bout with cancer and side effects made normal moments sometimes look suspicious. So, as she slid by, she asked, "Everything OK?"

I frowned and wondered if I should tell her. I didn't want to, didn't want to ruin this celebration. But I knew being honest was the right thing—the safe thing—to do, especially in the backcountry. Mary would have to deal with whatever happened; I should keep her informed.

"My vision just faded to gray," I said as matter-of-factly as possible.

"What?" She stopped a few yards in front of me and turned to face me. "Are you okay now?"

"I think so."

"Do you want to go on?"

I felt torn. I wanted to continue so we could have more time on this trail. But was that wise? "I'll go for a bit more, but I'm going to slow my pace."

"You sure?"

"Yeah," I said, feeling unsure.

"Please be careful." As she skied away, she yelled over her shoulder, "And we can turn around whenever you want."

I pulled my poles out of the snow and slid one ski in front of the other. I was slow at first, then a bit faster, but still slower than before things went wonky. My vision had returned to normal, but I felt very fatigued. I had to work hard to maintain a slow pace even when the climb wasn't steep. I knew Mary was dogging it so she wouldn't ski too far ahead. I appreciated her keeping me in sight.

After struggling for about another mile, I gave up. I stopped and yelled to her, "I want to go back now." I turned my skis downhill and waited for her. I felt embarrassed, but I sensed the return trip would be an energy challenge, even with the help of gravity.

"How do you feel right now?" Mary asked, sliding beside me.

"Exhausted."

"You want some water?"

That was a good idea. I should have thought of that. Was I not thinking clearly? I nodded, and she pulled the insulated bottle from my pack's side pouch. After I drank deeply, we began the descent to the car.

I sighed with fatigue even as gravity helped me move along. Keeping my body upright took more effort than usual. My hormone therapy and resulting low testosterone had probably helped create this moment. I had recently read studies that explained how fatigue increases as long-term hormone therapy continues—my eighteen months definitely qualified as long-term.

Even though treatment was about to end, the hormone that had been injected repeatedly to stop my body from producing testosterone would take months to leave. Meanwhile, low testosterone could create more moments like this.

Skiing in such frigid temperatures didn't help either. Given what I knew about low testosterone and its side effects, I felt like kicking myself for even being out there. But being out there was why we lived here.

I released a loud sigh of relief when we arrived back at the trailhead. We clicked out of our skis and slid them into the car. "I'll drive," Mary said.

I thanked her. She had driven to the trailhead, and we had planned for me to drive home. But with how I felt, I doubted that was safe. Obviously, she did, too.

I sank into the passenger seat. It felt great to sit still and guzzle water. Mary started driving and turned the heat on high. As the car warmed, my body tingled, this time with relief.

"Okay with you if I try to sleep?" I asked.

"Sure. Have a good nap."

I slid the seat back and pulled my wool hat over my eyes. I had wanted to celebrate the upcoming end of treatment and beginning of follow-up. But that ski was a scary reminder that it would take time—perhaps months—before my testosterone started to rebuild and my energy, strength, and endurance returned. This battle was far from over.

Though I wasn't celebrating, I had no regrets about choosing radiation and hormone therapy, even with all the troubling side effects. I felt proud that Mary and I had taken such an active role in my treatment — the first line of defense — and that we had developed our DARE approach as the second line.

And I felt determined that, no matter what happened, I would stay focused on diet, attitude, rest, and exercise while spending active and healing time in nature in this place I love.

CHAPTER 46

End of Treatment

Two weeks later, the end-of-treatment consult began with the oncologist clicking into the computer and saying, "So your testosterone is still low. In theory, that last injection should be expiring about now, but it's going to take two to six months for your testosterone [level] to come up."

Given that challenging ski, I expected that low testosterone level. When I asked what I could expect in terms of changes while the testosterone rose, he said that the first indication that testosterone was recovering would be a decrease in the frequency and intensity of the hot flashes. "The longer your testosterone is elevated, your stamina, your energy level, and your strength will improve."

That sounded good, but he hadn't mentioned the changes to our sex life, so I asked about erections and libido. "Libido will return when the testosterone comes back up. But that's separate from erections. The libido typically returns first, and then hopefully the erections will recover."

Hopefully? That left a lot to be desired, but I knew he was being honest with me. Moving on, I inquired about anemia, another side effect we had been monitoring. He pulled up the results of the day's blood work and stared at the screen. He scrolled through the iron studies and said he had no concerns about the results. He said I was not iron-deficient, and there was nothing I needed to change.

Finally, it was time to address the elephant in the room: the possibility of recurrence and spread. I asked his opinion based on the latest blood work. "I honestly can't tell you any more than when I first met you. The hormone therapy has been suppressing the PSA, and the effectiveness of the treatment is ultimately related to the radiation. But we don't know what the radiation has done until your testosterone recovers." Perhaps responding to my silence and frown, he added that he viewed the goal of the treatment as completely eradicating the cancer.

"So you want the treatment to be curative?" Mary chimed in.

"Correct. So you never have to deal with this again."

"How often do you achieve that?" I asked, afraid to hear his answer. When he replied that it depends on the PSA and biopsy results when treatment began, I reminded him that my original PSA was twenty-five, and the biopsy had found one very aggressive sample.

He clicked into his notes, started reading, and fell into a long silence. He released a big exhale, "I mean, I'd say you've probably got a seventy percent long-term cure rate."

Well, I thought, *my chance of recurrence just fell from fifty percent to thirty. That's good.*

I thanked him for the estimate and added that I would not hold him to it. I was just trying to figure out what was going on in my body. I explained that I would continue with the diet Mary and I had created. I would continue to focus on rest and exercise because I can control those areas while no longer in treatment. With or without cancer, focusing on diet, rest, and exercise would still help me.

He said that we will meet every three months until my testosterone increases. "And then, assuming the PSA is okay, then I stretch it out to every six months for a while."

I asked what changes in PSA would concern him. "What I would hope for is that it doesn't get above one. It should be very low." He added that when radiation oncologists debate what the definition of a recurrence should be, "it's if the PSA gets above two. But I like it to stay lower than that."

Mary asked his opinion on the doubling effect that we had read about.

"The doubling time comes into play," he said, "if we're convinced we have a recurrence, and then we're wondering how fast things are going." He said that if six months from now my PSA was two, he would be worried. If three months after that, it was six, he would see that as a fast doubling time and probably recommend a return to hormone therapy.

Mary asked whether there would be any long-term radiation effects. "We definitely have the effects during the treatment when we're acutely inflaming the bowel and the bladder," he said. When he added that he wouldn't expect my bowel or bladder function to get worse, I told him that was a relief.

He nodded and began shutting down the computer and the session. Time to give thanks.

"Coming in here to begin with," I said, "I was nervous as hell. You and the rest of your team have been so friendly and professional and skilled that I feel like I sailed through this, and I want to thank you for that."

He smiled and said, "You've been a pleasure to take care of." He added that he enjoys patients like Mary and me, who are interested in their health and ask good questions.

As I stood to shake his hand, the high achiever in me smiled and took a final bow.

CHAPTER 47

An End and a Beginning

FINALLY, THE TREATMENT LEG OF THE JOURNEY INTO THE wilds of cancer had ended. My very low PSA number showed the treatment had succeeded: if any cancer cells remained in my body, they were not active. That troublesome treatment to keep my aggressive cancer cells from killing me was worth the trouble.

As the forty-four shots of radiation killed cancer cells, they produced lots of gastrointestinal issues. Worth it.

As the eighteen months of hormone therapy lowered my testosterone levels and starved my cancer cells, they also brought me hot flashes, erectile dysfunction, loss of interest in sex, increasing fatigue, loss of muscle mass, and possible loss of bone density. Worth it.

Since diagnosis, while our skilled medical team went about their work of recommending and providing treatment, Mary and I spent hours, days, and weeks researching, formulating, and implementing DARE. Worth it.

For me, my low PSA number confirmed that incorporating DARE, along with conventional medical treatment—a medical and personal approach—helped the treatment succeed. As radiation and hormone therapy did their duty, our revised diet starved cancer cells and nurtured healthy cells. Sufficient rest provided my body, mind, and heart with the recovery each needed. Consistent exercise reduced stress, countered the side effects of treatment, and helped my body recover. A positive and hopeful outlook, along with time in nature, kept me in the fight. This approach took time, energy, and commitment. Worth it.

Beginning the next phase, follow-up and recovery, does not mean our battle has ended. I still have a thirty percent chance of recurrence, even though my oncologist's stated treatment goal was to kill every cancer cell in my body. There's no guarantee he succeeded—or failed. All we can do is monitor my PSA number and testosterone level during the months and years ahead. The two measures are intimately related and could present good news and bad news.

The good news: If my testosterone level rises, I should enjoy a decrease in side effects, although that may be tempered in a man my age.

The bad news: If my testosterone level rises and there are still prostate cancer cells in my body, those tough little testosterone-gobbling buggers could feast on that increasing supply and multiply. That could push my PSA higher, indicate a recurrence, and mean more treatment and more troubles.

But those are all unknowns, hidden dangers. Mary and I know we're not helpless as treatment ends. We have DARE, as well as time in nature, to continue working towards our overarching goal: to make my body a hostile environment for cancer cells and a haven for healthy cells. Diet, rest, and exercise can help increase my strength, energy, and endurance, while also reducing muscle loss and any bone density loss. Hopefully, my time biking, hiking, or skiing will not be tainted — as it was recently — with the scary need to cut that ski short and struggle back to the car. Only time will tell.

I have reached the desired destination on one leg of this journey into the wilds of cancer. This leg challenged my body, mind, and heart in ways I could never have imagined. Would not have wanted to imagine.

I have begun the next leg of this journey, follow-up and recovery. I'm hopeful and committed to working hard and making the life-affirming decisions needed to achieve a future free of prostate cancer.

A Message to the Reader

I chose to self-publish this book and my previous books because I wanted more control over the finished work. But self-publishing means that I don't have the muscle of a traditional publisher to promote the work and get it into the hands of interested readers. There's just me. And you, the satisfied reader.

You can help me — and other indie authors — by taking a moment to post a review and rating of this book on social media or wherever you bought the book. Your review helps other readers find books by indie authors.

Thanks for reading and helping,

Rick

I welcome readers to visit me on social media:

Substack: lamplugh.substack.com
Facebook: (@rick.lamplugh)
Bluesky (@ricklamplugh)
Vimeo (vimeo.com/ricklamplugh)

About the Author

For ten years, Rick Lamplugh lived in Gardiner, Montana, at Yellowstone National Park's north entrance. During that time, he wrote, spoke, and photographed to protect wildlife and preserve wild lands. He has since moved to Livingston, Montana, a beautiful fifty-two-mile drive from Yellowstone. Along with his address, his writing focus has also changed as he entered the wilds of aging and was later diagnosed with aggressive prostate cancer.

His last book, *The Wilds of Aging: A Journey of Heart and Mind*, won the National Indie Excellence Award. It was a finalist in the Next Generation Indie Book Awards. It won Honorable Mention in the Reader Views Literary Awards. As one reviewer wrote, "Rick beautifully weaves a deep love of the outdoors and nature into a poignant and tangible contemplation of aging. A wonderful and moving read."

The previous book, *Deep into Yellowstone: A Year's Immersion in Grandeur and Controversy,* won a Gold Medal in the Independent Publisher Book Awards. It was a finalist in the Next Generation Indie Book Awards and in the National Indie Excellence Awards. It won an Honorable Mention in the Eric Hoffer Book Awards and in the INDIES Book Awards. As one reviewer wrote, "A touch of

Bill Bryson's whimsy, a dose of Edward Abbey's insight, and the storytelling charm of John McPhee."

His earlier book, *In the Temple of Wolves: A Winter's Immersion in Wild Yellowstone,* was an Amazon best seller with more than five hundred Five-Star reviews. As one reviewer wrote, "Rich with facts on the Park and the wildlife that inhabit it, and deep with the feelings they inspire. Be prepared to laugh and cry, and to long for a visit – or another visit – to Yellowstone."

Rick's stories have appeared in the literary journals *Composite Arts Magazine, Gold Man Review, Phoebe, Soundings Review,* and *Feathered Flounder.* He won the Jim Stone Grand Prize for Non-Fiction.

Acknowledgments

From diagnosis, through treatment, and into recovery, I saw many medical professionals. Three provided the conventional medical treatment that worked well for me. My thanks to Nicole Bressler, DO, Daniel Swanson, MD, and David Koeplin, MD. Two other providers were helpful in my treatment, but in a different way. Noelle Butler, ND, and Kendall Child, NP, took extra time to listen, share, and educate. I thank them both.

The radiation team, nurses, and aides at Bozeman Health Cancer Center were efficient and effective, while friendly and supportive. So was the front desk staff. That combination made going in for treatment a pleasure, even when I dreaded the treatment side effects.

All these professionals not only provided excellent medical care but also encouraged and supported me, sometimes with words, sometimes with smiles. They provided the first line of defense. And succeeded!

I want to express my gratitude to all the men I met in the waiting room at the Cancer Center. Once I pushed myself to open up and ask questions, I had conversations with many who helped me understand cancer and endure months of treatment.

I also pushed myself to reach out to other men I knew in search of deeper sharing. Thank you, Dan Shapiro, Jim Good, John Swanson, Wolfgang Dengler, Kim Johansen, Arnie Schuster, John Costello, and Leo Leckie, for the time, thoughts, and feelings you shared.

Another source of support was the Cancer Support Community Montana. Through that organization, I attended weekly Zoom workout sessions led by a trainer who kept me moving, even when I was deep into treatment and didn't feel like exercising. I also attended a monthly men's support group with a facilitator who kept me and other cancer patients talking and supporting each other.

My active friends—partners in hikes, walks, and cross-country skiing—supported me as I slowed down due to treatment-induced fatigue. My time in nature with them was healing at whatever pace we took. Thank you, Julianne Baker, Fred Baker, Diane Renkin, Jane Olsen, Patty Walton, Woody Martyn, Betty Martyn, and Leo Leckie.

A special thanks to Jeanne Holmes for sharing her experience with handling a life-changing illness. Greg Field, another man with prostate cancer, also shared much about his battle.

The chapters in this book, like the chapters in my previous books, began with honest sharing with my paper therapist. When that sharing raised questions, I researched them and added the findings to the chapter. Thanks, in particular, to the Prostate Cancer Foundation and Active Surveillance Patients International. Both organizations provided significant, accurate, and helpful information about prostate cancer treatment and recovery.

After completing the research, I edited the chapters to combine storytelling with science. Once comfortable with the results, I wanted to hear what readers thought.

Early on, I sent the first two chapters to friends. The comments of Woody Martyn, Betty Martyn, Bill Ripple, Tom Titus, Tajali Tolan, Vicki Sielaf, and Fred Baker encouraged me to keep going. Thanks to each of you.

As treatment progressed and I added more chapters, I created a Substack titled *The Wilds of Cancer*. There, I posted preview chapters to see how readers I didn't know responded. I thank all those folks who not only read the chapters but also took the time to offer supportive and helpful comments. I extend special thanks to the readers who kindly permitted me to use their names and comments on the "What Readers Say" pages at the front of this book. I also thank the helping professionals who took time from their busy schedules to read the final manuscript and write a blurb.

My family was a huge help in this battle. They were willing to ask me how I was doing and to listen and respond. Their loving hugs and words helped me refocus on the battle, even when I felt I couldn't go on. My love and thanks to Allison, Zack, Hana, Siena, Rus, Judy, Alan, Clara, Jim, and Janet.

And then there's Mary, a cancer survivor and caregiver beyond belief. From the moment of diagnosis, through months of troubling treatment and recovery, this dedicated partner lovingly changed her life to help me save mine. I could not have done this without Mary. I love her dearly and will be forever grateful.

An Excerpt from

The Wilds of Aging:
A Journey of Heart and Mind

CHAPTER 1

The North Cascades

Without expecting to, I began my journey into the wilds of aging during a two-week-long, 375-mile bicycle tour at age sixty. I rode alone, lugging a fifty-pound trailer stuffed with camping gear up and down the mountains of Washington's North Cascades in July.

I don't usually tour alone, but one of my riding partners, my wife, Mary, had to work. My other riding partner, Jim, had to drop out just after he and I had finished making the plans and preparations for the tour. I decided to go solo, even though doing so made me nervous: I would have no one with whom to share the daily challenges of a long ride in mountainous, unfamiliar territory, no one to encourage or be encouraged by.

But the challenges of this long tour also excited me. I enjoy adventuring and pushing myself. During each of the seven previous summers, Mary and I had completed weeks-long adventures—biking or hiking—that we designed to stretch ourselves physically, mentally, and emotionally. We pedaled long, self-supported bike rides in mountains and deserts in our home state of Oregon. We hiked deep into the wild backcountry of Yellowstone and Glacier National Parks. We struggled side by side up mountains in the West and in Maine.

So there I was, halfway into the North Cascades tour, alone and cooking in full sun as I cycled up a steep road in a canyon scented by the hot lodgepole pines that dotted its sunbaked walls. Occasionally, a few pines shaded the road, but I passed through the shade far too quickly. The temperature broke ninety degrees before noon. The air rising from the blacktop was surely hotter.

The grade showed no sign of ending, and that oven of a road was challenging me like nothing had before. Even though I alternated standing and sitting as I pedaled, my legs grew limp and my pedaling slowed. But I kept pushing—and nervously glancing at the heart rate monitor on my sports watch. As the beats-per-minute number climbed, I fantasized the monitor would soon flash 9-1-1. And I was way out of cell phone range.

As the day burned on, the distance between breaks grew shorter. Each time I stopped, I forced myself to drink the now-hot—not just warm—water I carried. Finally, I heard the call of rushing water and pulled off the road.

I dismounted and picked my way rock by rock down a steep bank to an enticing stream. I knelt, dunked my head completely into the cold water, and kept it there until I ran out of air. I jerked my head out of the water and shook it like a wet dog would. Gasping, I lay back on a hot rock and proclaimed to the empty sky, "That's it. I've hit my limit." The confession surprised me: that was the first time I had ever admitted reaching a physical limit.

I wanted to believe that the problem was just the hill, the heat, the hour, nothing I couldn't overcome. But lying there, feeling the sun vaporize water off my face, I wasn't so sure. I even wondered if pushing on might be dangerous. What if I passed out while cycling alone on this little-used mountain road?

Still, I had miles to go before making camp, and introspection — or lying on that rock and drinking that stream dry — wouldn't get me there. I stripped off my sweat-stained, yellow biking shirt and submerged it in the creek. Not bothering to wring it out, I pulled it on and shivered as if I had just jumped into the stream.

I climbed up the bank to my bike and looked ahead. I faced many switchbacks; each would bring me closer to my next goal, mile-high Washington Pass, up there in the conifers and flanked by ragged mountain peaks. I shook my head at the elevation and distance yet to cover. Then I mounted up, gritted my teeth, and pedaled on.

I made it to the pass and down the other side, and eventually reached camp. When I finally stepped off my bike, I stumbled, exhausted, to the site's picnic table. I looked at the fire pit but knew there would be no camp-fire for me. I would just eat, set up my tent, and lay my tired old body down.

Several days later, I finished the tour, but the memory of reaching my limit that day stuck in my craw. Once back home, I told Jim, who is four years older than I, and Mary, who is four years younger, how I had reached my limit and how much that bothered me. They both said I'd get over it.

That sounded good. But I doubted it.

CHAPTER 2

South Sister

A MONTH AFTER THAT SOLO BIKE TOUR, MARY AND I stepped out of our tent at three in the morning to start a climb of 10,358-foot South Sister in Oregon's Cascades. We chattered with energy and excitement, awed by the otherworldly glow of our headlamps' beams glittering off a white gravel trail. We weren't expecting a tough hike; this route is a "walk-up" that thousands of people attempt each year, and most make it. We were climbing as a warm-up for a higher—and more challenging—peak in Wyoming later in the summer.

As the day wore on and we climbed above tree line, my energy and excitement wore out. I struggled on in fits and starts, heart pounding, thighs burning. My breaks grew longer and more frequent, just as they had in the North Cascades.

On one break, I turned and gazed downhill. Below me, Mary moved slowly but steadily up the mountain in what she calls "chug mode." Watching her patient progress, I caught myself trying to convince myself that I had gone far enough. That the smart move was to quit pushing, turn around, and cruise downhill. That I had nothing to prove. That I wasn't a failure.

I shook off these thoughts and moved on. Rounding a corner, I came upon the start of a mile-long, steeper section of loose, rough, red volcanic rock that we would have to slip and slide up to reach the now-visible summit. Two young men sat comfortably beside the trail.

I stopped and asked, "Are you going for the summit?"

One of the young men, hood up, arms across his chest, shook his head and answered, "No, I'm not going any farther."

Projecting that he might be struggling, as I was, with feeling like a failure, I encouraged him to go on.

There was a moment of silence, and then the second young man looked at me, smiled, and said, "I've never climbed a mountain before, and I'm happy to have gotten this high. I think I'll stop right here, too."

I glanced down the trail and saw Mary, still out of earshot. I turned to the young men and complimented them on knowing their limits. Then I said, "I don't know how many more mountains I have inside me." I felt surprised at telling two strangers something I had never told anyone, not even myself. They nodded silently. I nodded back.

I walked ahead a few paces and waited for Mary. Together, she and I climbed on, challenging and encouraging one another as we had done on so many other hikes. When we finally stepped hand in hand onto the summit of South Sister, I knew — as I had on that solo bike tour — that I had reached a physical limit. As I gazed down the mountain to where the young men had accepted their limits, reaching this summit felt like senseless suffering, not the grand accomplishment I had hoped for.

After slogging back to base camp, Mary and I sat on a fallen log and watched late afternoon thunderheads form. As the clouds rumbled our way, we retreated to the tent. While Mary napped, I lay on my back, tired but unable to sleep. Hands locked behind my head, I stared at the tent ceiling. I thought about my last two outings—one solo, one not—and how I had reached the limit of my endurance and questioned the value of pushing on.

Lightning cracked, thunder boomed, and the mountains echoed. I curled up into the protection of my sleeping bag and realized there was more: I had confessed to the young men that I didn't know how many more mountains I could tackle. That statement revealed something that should have been obvious long ago: aging and declining physical abilities could kill the adventuring I so loved. Worse yet, aging would eventually kill me.

I watched drops of rain land on the tent fly, join into rivulets, and slide downward, pushing dust ahead. Of course I was aging; everyone ages—if they're lucky. And everyone dies—lucky or not. The real wonder was that I had denied these ancient and obvious truths for so long. How had I managed to maintain, like Peter Pan, an illusion of unending youth?

CHAPTER 3

The Wall

PRESERVING THAT ILLUSION HAD REQUIRED ME TO BUILD a wall around myself, a wall that blocked thoughts of my mortality, a wall so strong that even at sixty years of age I had not accepted the reality of aging. But that South Sister climb and the North Cascades bike tour had proved to me that, regardless of what I'm willing to admit, my body is aging, and aging leads to physical decline and eventually death.

I started building that protective wall a decade earlier when Jana, our friend of eighteen years, died from cancer. She was younger than me and my equal in the way she challenged and cared for her athletic body. If she couldn't beat death, I wondered then, how could I? That glimpse of a terrible truth threatened my illusion of unending youth. I mixed a big batch of denial and started building. The wall wasn't big or strong, but it would have to do.

Five years after Jana's passing, our friend Daniel was diagnosed with ALS. He asked Mary, me, and a couple of other close friends to help him on his final journey. During his last year, each time we sadly watched him lose the ability to bicycle, hike, and climb, I glimpsed the truth: If death could steal Daniel's joys, couldn't it steal mine?

That took a wrecking ball to the wall. With squeals and groans, chunks tumbled down, littering my inner landscape. When the dust settled, there were still scattered remnants to hide behind. But everywhere else, the truth of aging, declining, and dying shattered my illusion and scared me. I mixed up more denial and started patching.

Three years after Daniel's death, Misty, one of the first people to befriend us when we moved to Oregon many years ago, was diagnosed with cancer for the second time and told this was a battle she couldn't win. An experienced hospice worker, she took the time to prepare her memorial service, start to finish. After Mary and I attended that touching service, I sensed that preparing my memorial service might ease my fears — if I stopped denying and started planning. A big if.

The same year Misty died, my brother, sister, and I moved our mother into a Delaware nursing home. As she has descended into the abyss of Alzheimer's, I have watched her memories depart, her personhood pass away. This leaves me frightened that I will follow her forgetful footsteps.

The deaths of Jana, Daniel, and Misty pounded the point home: I will die. Each cross-country visit to Mom — three or four times a year — left me feeling that I was watching a painful preview of how death might take me. Scared and vulnerable, I took shelter behind the wall, clung to the illusion, acted as if nothing had changed. Until the summer that began with the exhausting North Cascades bike tour and the draining climb of South Sister.

That summer ended with a three-week adventure that began with a backpack trip deep into Wyoming's Wind River Range to climb that higher peak that we hoped South Sister had prepared us for. But hikers and stock trains, horses carrying riders and mules carrying cargo, crowded the trail we had to take to reach the base of the mountain. We managed to ignore the sight, sound, and smell of the multitude of trail users until we rounded a corner and came upon a dead pinto packhorse, swollen, stinking, and stiff-legged, beside the trail.

Hand over her nose, Mary said, "What in the world is that doing there?"

I shook my head in disbelief and said, "You got me."

"Are they just going to leave it there?"

"Well, I've heard that they sometimes remove dead stock in a sling under a helicopter. Or if that doesn't work, they blow it up."

"Blow it up? That's unbelievable," Mary said with disgust. "Let's get off this trail and find something resembling wilderness."

With the pain of climbing South Sister fresh in my mind, I readily agreed to leave the trail and forgo the higher peak. We bushwhacked off trail and found an isolated spot barely big enough for our tent but overlooking an absolute gem of a lake.

We made ourselves a home, and for each of the next three days, we strolled the short distance from the campsite to the lake. There we played in the water, sunned ourselves on hot rocks, watched wildlife, and listened to the wind. I actually enjoyed *not* challenging myself. I loved *sitting still*! What was wrong with me?

After a few restful days, we packed out and drove north to Yellowstone and the next adventure. Several days into the backcountry, I sat in soothing shade along-side murmuring Coyote Creek, its streambed decorated with red and gold pebbles, tumbled smooth. I confessed to my journal that I feared the worst fate I could then imagine: turning into an old man who hears about others challenging themselves and mutters, "I used to do that."

At the end of our hike, Mary and I checked into a motel and stayed for the first time in Gardiner, Montana, at Yellowstone's north gate. After a good night's sleep, we took the steps from the motel down to a wooden deck thirty feet above the Yellowstone River. Off to our right, faint early-morning light kissed Electric Peak and turned the sky a purplish blue. The white noise of the river drowned all sound of the town's awakening. Mary, her face red from windburn, sat on a step adjusting our camp stove, adding the aroma of coffee to the sage-scented air as the last day of our summer adventure began.

As I admired the high-desert landscape, the light swelled, transforming the river from black to dark green to aqua, decorated with white caps and lighter green tongues and chutes. High clouds above Electric Peak glowed tangerine.

Watching the light change, I thought about how I had changed over the summer. Physically, my endurance for rigorous adventures had faded. Mentally, my confidence had wavered. Emotionally, frustration and fears now abounded.

I didn't share these scary revelations with Mary. I wasn't ready to accept them myself. What I didn't know then was how much more I had yet to face and accept in the wilds of aging.